What People Are Sayi[ng]
Andrew Butterworth and *I'm Si[ck]*...

Dr. Andrew Butterworth has written a very helpful, practical, balanced book on healing. I believe *I'm Sick Now What?* will be a great blessing to those in need of healing and to those who are praying and caring for loved ones with sickness. It is filled with great insight from a pastor who has been a medical doctor. I recommend *I'm Sick Now What?* to you as one of the important books on healing you should have in your library.

—*Dr. Randy Clark*
Founder of Global Awakening
www.globalawakening.com

Finally, a balanced, well-rounded book on healing. *I'm Sick, Now What?* covers the major questions that Christians ask about healing and health. This book is theologically sound, intellectually stimulating, and user-friendly. If you have questions about healing as a Christian, read this book!

—*Steve Murrell*
Cofounder, Every Nation
www.everynation.org
www.stevemurrell.com

Andrew trained as a medical doctor and now works on the pastoral staff of a local church. His unique position is the soil from which this book has grown, with its unique and fully-orbed view of healing. He covers the medical, emotional, spiritual, and theological aspects of healing with thoughtful care. Personally, I have been waiting for a hybrid book on physical healing that calls for personal responsibility in one's physical and emotional health, while still having a theology and expectancy for Jesus to heal. This is that book! May it take root and bear fruit for the good of many and for the glory of God. I commend it to you.

—*Alan Frow*
Lead pastor, Southlands Church, California
www.southlands.net

Finally, a book that combines faith for holistic healing through supernatural means as well as healing through medical means. It's not only theologically sound, but pastorally-minded. It helps to answer our questions when God doesn't heal. I can't wait to get this into the hands of our church members.

—*Bryan Mowrey*
Lead pastor, Jubilee Church, St. Louis, Missouri
www.jubileestl.org

Dr. Butterworth's book is clear, concise, and heartening. He deals with a very sensitive topic in a way that is both encouraging and informative. Take it from someone who has experienced both illness (myeloproliferative disorder) and healing (bone marrow transplant), if there's one book you should read on illness and healing, it's this one.

—*Darryn Botha*
Lead pastor, Cape Town Baptist Church,
Cape Town, South Africa

I'm Sick, Now What? is a balanced examination of healing by a physician-pastor, Dr. Andrew Butterworth, whose name tag should read, "soul doctor." Unlike authors who address the question of healing from a purely physical perspective, dismissing the supernatural, or from a purely metaphysical perspective, dismissing the role of modern medicine, Dr. Butterworth's advice is to seek and employ the best of both, since all truth is from God, and only the truth can set you free. The author is uniquely trained and positioned to address questions related to illness, from a medically infused biblical perspective. Anyone who is sick and wants to know how to approach their illness can benefit from this book.

—*David B. Biebel, DMin*
Author, editor, publisher
Healthy Life Press
www.healthylifepress.com

Based firmly on biblical truth and years of medical knowledge as a doctor, a hugely practical book. It gives clear guidelines on how to connect deeply with our loving Father God, remove the blockages that may be standing in the way of healing, and pray for healing. It is full of testimonies of supernatural healing as well as healing through the medical profession. Andrew helpfully reminds us, however, that God is primarily interested in our coming to wholeness and fullness of life in Him. He speaks of the holistic health of spirit, soul, and body, which we can find in Him despite and even through physical ailments. I have no doubt that the prophecy spoken over Andrew years ago will be fulfilled and that many will find health and wholeness through this book.

—*Steve Goss*
International Director, Freedom In Christ Ministries
www.ficminternational.org

Andrew was at our house on the day I was diagnosed with cancer and throughout my ordeal was excellent friend, counselor, and doctor. This book is a great blend of spiritual, medical, and practical wisdom concerning sickness and healing.

—*PJ Smyth*
Founder, GodFirst, Johannesburg, South Africa
Leader of Advance, a worldwide church planting network
www.advancemovement.com

A pastoral, practical, sensible, and inspiring guide to healing that moves the heart, instructs the mind, and lifts faith by repeatedly pointing the reader to Jesus. For a topic that sometimes is beset by the extremes of either unreal triumphalism or faithless fatalism, Dr. Butterworth instead teaches a biblical and expectant realism—that the Divine Healer from Galilee is still walking through our towns and cities and is healing through the church and through the medical professions, daily. The writing style is accessible, engaging, and educational, the stories moving, and the teaching biblically as well as medically informed. I do not know of another book like it and warmly commend it to all who want to understand healing, as well as grow in practicing this vitally important aspect of the church's mission.

—*Dr. Adam Dodds*
Senior pastor, Elim Church, Dunedin, New Zealand
dunedin.elim.org.nz

I have come to know Andrew not only as a co-laborer in the gospel, but as a friend, now an author, and most profoundly as one who lives what he believes. He has prayed for my son who was instantly and supernaturally healed of an illness he battled for months but on another occasion, when he hosted me on a ministry trip and I was ill, he provided me with medication. As you read *I'm Sick, Now What?*, you will find, as I have, that Andrew does not shy away from the difficult questions but rather takes them head on and provides deep and meaningful insights. I have no doubt you will find your paradigms being challenged while discovering handles to experiencing God's unfailing love even when our experiences don't make sense.

—*Frans Olivier*
Senior pastor, Every Nation Church, Nairobi, Kenya
Senior evangelist, Every Nation Southern Africa

Andrew has written a book which I feel will be tremendously helpful to all believers. As a pastor, I see the value of this book in helping people understand and process illness, pain, and disappointment while encouraging them to seek God's loving hand for healing. The strength of this book is its balance and its breadth, including biblical teaching, pastoral sensitivity, medical experience, and many stories of real life. All of this is portrayed with a tender heart desirous of people coming to real wholeness, which is God's heart. I would highly recommend this very thorough and engaging book.

—*Wayne Noland*,
Lead elder/pastor, The Rock Christian Church,
Cape Town, South Africa
www.therockcc.org.za

In this book, Andrew Butterworth shows how medical science sits comfortably within a biblical Christian worldview. His accessible writing style and compelling personal stories make it a must-read for anyone looking for answers to some of life's most painful questions.

—*Sibs Sibanda*
Lead pastor, City Hill Church, Johannesburg, South Africa
www.cityhillchurch.org.za

Dr. Andrew Butterworth has not written a typical "rise and be healed" scenario, but rather a deeply contemplative and extremely well-proportioned insight and prognosis into the very heart of God when it comes to healthy lives. This needs to be a best-seller around the world and read by everyone who desires a thorough understanding of how to deal with the inner conflicts of mankind.

—*Philip DeVries*
CEO, EDEN Leadership Foundation
www.edenleadership.com

In this excellent book, Dr. Andrew Butterworth presents a fascinating set of answers to the problem of sickness. As a trained medical doctor and a pastor of a church, Dr. Butterworth straddles both realms seamlessly. He opens the door for those who have hitherto only considered natural means of healing to venture into the much wider and richer world of the Spirit—while those who have been solely involved with the spiritual world are enriched with wisdom from the natural world. Dr. Butterworth draws very valuable insights that show us that healing from God is not only accessible but also quite a practical matter. He takes us beyond the "how to" of healing and helps us to meet with *Yahweh Rophe*, "the God Who Heals." I predict that many shall be healed through reading this book, and many more shall be stirred and empowered to bring God's healing to all who are sick.

—*Dr. John Kpikpi*
Senior pastor, City of God Church, Accra, Ghana
www.cityofgodchurch.net

I'M SICK

NOW WHAT?

DR. ANDREW BUTTERWORTH

WHITAKER
HOUSE

Unless otherwise indicated, all Scripture quotations are taken from *The Holy Bible, English Standard Version*, © 2000, 2001, 1995 by Crossway Bibles, a division of Good News Publishers. Used by permission. All rights reserved. Scripture quotations marked (NIV) are taken from the *Holy Bible, New International Version*®, NIV®, © 1973, 1978, 1984 by Biblica, Inc.® Used by permission. All rights reserved worldwide.

Boldface type in the Scripture quotations indicates the author's emphasis.

I'm Sick, Now What?
A Balanced Approach to Medicine and God's Healing

Andrew Butterworth
info@drandrewbutterworth.com
www.drandrewbutterworth.com

ISBN: 978-1-62911-561-0
eBook ISBN: 978-1-62911-583-2
Printed in the United States of America
© 2015 by Andrew Butterworth

Whitaker House
1030 Hunt Valley Circle
New Kensington, PA 15068
www.whitakerhouse.com

Library of Congress Cataloging-in-Publication Data
Butterworth, Andrew, 1980–
 I'm sick, now what? : a balanced approach to medicine and God's healing / Dr. Andrew Butterworth, BMedSc, MBChB, MRes (Public Health).
  pages cm
 ISBN 978-1-62911-561-0 (trade pbk. : alk. paper) — ISBN 978-1-62911-583-2
(ebook : alk. paper) 1. Healing—Religious aspects—Christianity. 2. Spiritual healing.
3. Medicine—Religious aspects—Christianity. I. Title.
BT732.B88 2015
261.5′61—dc23
       2015028393

1 2 3 4 5 6 7 8 9 10 11 **W** 22 21 20 19 18 17 16 15

To Michelle,

"I have set you as a seal upon my heart,
as a seal upon my arm
for love is strong as death,
jealously is fierce as the grave...
many waters cannot quench love."

(Song of Solomon 8:6 paraphrase)

CONTENTS

PREFACE

As a pastor, I have books I can recommend on relationships, marriage, parenting, and so on. But when someone or someone's loved one falls ill, I don't have a good book that I can recommend. The books I knew of in this area either focus on teaching healthy people how to pray for the sick, or focus on how to help a sick person process why such bad things as sickness happen. The small selection of books I came across that were targeted at helping a person seek healing tended to be quite narrow and built people up to expect supernatural healing automatically; if the person was in the difficult emotional place of seeking supernatural healing and not receiving it, however, the books had no helpful guidance.

As a trained medical doctor, I needed a book that wouldn't dismiss God's wisdom in modern medicine but as a believer, I needed a book that also wouldn't discard the concept of divine healing. And it needed to be a book that left people in a better place after reading it than before they started it. While I was still being trained as a doctor, a pastor had told me that he thought I would be a spiritual doctor one day and that I would write such a book that would enable people to access healing from God.

Many years later, here it is.

I write from a Christian worldview, but this book is written for everyone and anyone. A few years back, some British doctors went to China to evaluate traditional Chinese medicine from a Western perspective. They were told that the Chinese practitioners would happily explain their system of medicine, but they would need to start by explaining the Buddhist principles that underlined it. Similarly, to understand Christian healing and health, you need to have a grasp of the underlying Christian principles. I will explain these principles, using biblical references, as we go along. If you are open to this process, then you should find the book to very informative and enjoyable, even if you do not always agree with my conclusions.

I have divided the book in three sections. Section one explains why there is sickness in the world. Section two identifies things that can hinder health and healing, while also blocking us from connecting to God. Finally, section three explores how to approach God for healing, whether through conventional or supernatural means.

For ease of language, throughout the book I use the word "sickness" as a generic term to cover illnesses, diseases, disabilities, etc. In this book I give a lot of knowledge from current medical research and show how this confirms the wisdom placed in the Bible in the area of healing. Knowledge is very important, and Jesus said that *"you will know the truth, and the truth that will set you free"* (John 8:32). However, knowledge needs to sink deep into us, descending from our head to our heart to bring true freedom, and this is best done through putting the knowledge we receive into practice. That's why I'd encourage you to also participate in the practical sections of the book.

Through following the principles in this book, my prayer is that God will give you the wisdom needed to access healing. This may be through leading you to the right healthcare professional, medication, or intervention, but it might also be through God supernaturally initiating healing in you. Some people reading this may receive a deep spiritual or emotional healing, and, if the vision shared by the pastor who prophesied over me is to be fulfilled, others will receive physical healing through reading this.

Either way, can I encourage you to be expectant as you read?

ACKNOWLEDGMENTS

Writing a book is a surprisingly big task and I am grateful to all the people who said yes when I came to them asking them for assistance.

John Kpikpi, Malcolm Gamon, Pete Kropman, and Chris Appel reviewed my original proposal and ensured that it was in a state to submit to a publisher. I am grateful for their honesty in the early drafts that vastly improved it. Having published previously, John was particularly encouraging to me. My fellow pastors at Junction Church gave much encouragement; Craig Elliott was particularly helpful as a sounding board for ideas and theological concepts throughout the whole project. Christie Sainsbury proofread the initial proposal and ensured the grammar and syntax were to a high standard.

I am thankful for Les Stobbe who agreed to represent me and I am grateful for all at Whitaker House who agreed to take me on as an author, even when I was living on the other side of the world. In particular, I am grateful to work with such a great editor at Whitaker House, Judith Dinsmore, who increased the readability and flow of the book. Sibs Sibanda cast his penetrating eye of a couple of the chapters and Glenn Nesbitt, from Johannesburg Bible College, corresponded back and forth, giving up a lot of his time to read the whole manuscript and ensure that my arguments had a good logical flow and that they were framed with the appropriate theological terminology, even if our views differed slightly.

Liz East gave input for the middle section, drawing on her vast counselling experience, which I am very grateful for. Wayne Noland corrected a number of references and gave great pastoral perspective. Rob Grant, with some assistance from Andrew Badham, chased up the facts of my stories, ensuring things are as accurate as possible. It is common at this point for authors to state that the final responsibility rests with them for accuracy, which is true, but if you do find any errors please inform me so that I can personally have a dig at these two great guys.

My parents John and Jan Butterworth read the entire manuscript and as well as being very encouraging, gave crucial feedback that has made it a much better book than it might have been. Eighty years plus (between them) of reading (and my Dad publishing) Christian books turned them into a great focus group. Jennie Wegerle kindly offered to edit the whole manuscript prior to it going to the publisher. While she has a superb eye for detail and a passion for accurate grammar, she is wise enough to know that syntax and grammar are there to serve the flow and pace of the writing and not obstruct it. I am grateful for the many hours she put in to this endeavor in support of the book.

I love testimonies and stories, and I have put many in to the book. Consequently I am thoroughly grateful to all the people I am friends with, or have ministered to, who gave me permission to include their stories. All their stories are true, but for people's privacy I have often used different names when telling the stories. I am also grateful for all the people who placed their stories in the public domain. Stories that testify to God's goodness are a blessing to the worldwide church, and I trust their inclusion here will also be considered a blessing.

I also want to thank Michelle, my beautiful wife, for her encouragement and support and for allowing me time late at night to write for months on end. Our daughter Pippa was sometimes my writing companion while she was settling into her routine, and she often made it easy to continue writing. In contrast, her brother, JJ, took a big interest in my keyboard and I am grateful that he didn't insert too much text. I am blessed to have such a wonderful family.

Finally, I want to thank God, who is the kindest Being in the universe. I still find it so wonderful that He is interested in the minutiae of my life and that I get to interact with Him and partner with Him. The good news of Jesus is still the most staggering thing ever, and I am looking forward to growing in the knowledge of it, (and the resultant friendship that has come out of it) during every passing year.

This book wouldn't have come about if God didn't initiate it and then line up all the right things to assist and shape it. I trust that He will ensure it be helpful to some of the many people in the world who are experiencing sickness. *Soli Deo Gloria.*

SECTION ONE:

UNDERSTANDING SICKNESS

"Health is not valued till sickness comes."
—*Thomas Fuller*
Seventeenth-century English vicar

"Scripture presents suffering both as necessary, because
of living in a fallen world, and tragic, because suffering is
not the way it is supposed to be."
—*Dr. Gregg Allison*
Twenty-first-century American theologian

"Those who dive in the sea of affliction bring up rare pearls."
—*Charles Spurgeon*
Renowned nineteenth-century British pastor

CHAPTER 1:

I'VE GOT QUESTIONS

"We are all ill: but even a universal sickness implies
an idea of health."
—*Lionel Trilling*
Twentieth-century American critic

It was meant to be a joyful moment. The doctor teased out the baby, expecting that in a few moments his first cry would ring out, bringing relief to the room and signifying that all was well. But it didn't happen. The baby opened his eyes and seemed to stare straight into mine for a few penetrating seconds. I watched the life drain out of him—as suddenly as somebody pulling a plug. It was harrowing! I was twenty years old, on a five-week missions trip around Uganda to see if I wanted to spend my life abroad as a missionary doctor. The mother of the child must have come in from the rural areas to give birth at the kindly Church of Uganda Hospital; being from a rural area, she had not been scanned, so nobody was prepared for what was about to happen. Her child was born with an extremely rare condition called anencephaly, a condition where the top of the head fails to form fully. This little baby had enough brain formation to keep him going in the womb, but as soon as he reached the outside world, the parts of the brain that needed to kick into gear to initiate breathing, etc., just weren't there.

As his tiny, blood-stained body went limp I felt the emotion in the room hit me—the initial tension of the delivery, the joy as the birth occurred, and then the gradual realization by everyone present that the baby, who a few moments before had been absorbing the world around him, had, just as quickly, passed away.

I didn't speak to many people that day. That was the first time I'd witnessed a death—and it was a little newborn, no less. My head was spinning with questions and my heart was aching with different emotions.

Years later I would find myself repeatedly being part of the team that delivered such bad news: "I am sorry, Mr. Martin, but the news is not what you wanted to hear. The sample of tissue came back from the lab and showed abnormal growth. I am sorry to say it is cancerous and it is very advanced." Or, "I am sorry to say that your brother has passed away." A few sentences that would send people's worlds spinning. Shock, anger, feelings of betrayal. Maybe you have experienced some of these feelings of confusion or despair, injustice or unfairness.

Sickness seems to have the power to bring out the most vulnerable part of us.

Just before I got married to my wife Michelle, I rented a room in the house of a family. The father was very successful in his industry, a brilliant public speaker, and always very confident and warm toward his staff. But, during my short stay, he was diagnosed with cancer and did not know whether he would live to see his children grow up. Michelle and I had heard the news from others and decided to see how the family was doing. We tentatively knocked on the door to the lounge, where they were all gathered watching TV, and were beckoned in. After muted hellos we tried to ask the most sensitive questions we could, but it was still so raw that as they answered our questions, the family started to cry, and soon our tears were falling to the floor too. Our limited grasp of the pain they were experiencing was communicated far better through tears than through our awkward attempts to ask questions moments earlier.

Probably the earliest-written book of the Bible tells the story of a man called Job who experienced terrible suffering, culminating in agonizing, total-body sores. In the narrative, three of his friends turned up after hearing the news and for seven whole days they sat in silence—not saying a word but deeply connecting with his suffering. Wisely, they knew this wasn't the time to try and puzzle what had gone wrong, nor the time to exhort him to have faith. These three friends had lived long enough to know that well-meaning words said in the wrong moment can come across as unloving or even harsh, and that good advice unsolicited is rarely heard. If you are familiar with the story you'll know that after that great start, Job's friends became more of a hindrance than a help, and their words caused more frustration than blessing. But their initial empathetic silence was very helpful; and after the week-long time of processing, Job was ready to make sense of the swirling questions and search for answers.

All of us reach that point eventually. It's only natural to want to have answers. We may, like Job, get frustrated and despondent if we don't seem to find the answers initially—if the people we go to don't seem to understand the problem or give us passionate answers that don't seem to resonate with our situation. But that doesn't mean the desire for answers has gone away.

Through my time as a medical doctor and lately as a full-time pastor, I have discovered that there are answers to be found. They might not be the answers we expect, but just as God engaged with Job, He will engage with us—He doesn't show partiality.[1] But God also showed Job that there are no quick fixes to pain; no satisfying pat answers or fortune cookie wisdom. What Job did find out

---

1. See Romans 2:11; Ephesians 6:9; Acts 10:34.

was that his deepest need for answers was met through a relationship. As another biblical patriarch, Jacob, found out years later, it is through the pursuit of God, not the fleeing from God, that God speaks; through the wrestling and not the withdrawing that God interacts. Both Job and Jacob got more than they expected, but they also got exactly what they needed. If there is anyone who knows what you need in your specific situation, anyone who understands where you are in the journey and what will help at each point along the way, it is God.

The tragedy today is that, often, our view of God has been tainted by negative experiences. We may have had a bad experience with father figures, making it difficult to relate to God as Father. A good friend may have betrayed us, and somehow the concept of Jesus being a Friend who's closer than a brother doesn't sound too attractive anymore. Or someone who was a comfort to us growing up may appear cold toward us now, making it harder to connect to the Holy Spirit as our Comforter.

In any relationship, if we pick up an inaccurate view of the other person, it can create a wedge. Have you ever had those moments where you thought somebody was being unkind toward you only to realize later that you completely misread the situation? If your experiences in life have made it difficult to think of God as utterly loving, then you might find it difficult to connect with Him during dark times. Maybe you read those sentences a couple of paragraphs back about God not showing partiality and thought, *He certainly loves me less—look at my situation compared to what He does for so and so.* But you may be misreading the situation. God said He shows no partiality, and if He really is God, then what He says is true.

Can there be a way to make sense of the situations we find ourselves in? What is God's view on sickness? Is healing possible? Is it possible for me? Does God want me to seek healing?

If the time is right for you—if you have reached the place that Job did and you want to make sense of the questions you have, then perhaps you will be willing to explore these questions with me. As a fellow journeyer, I cannot promise answers to everything, but I can show you what I have discovered, as I've seen times of magnificent victory and times of seemingly devastating defeat, as I've wept and cried with those who have lost relatives, and as I've danced with joy as God broke through miraculously.

It had been an exciting day. After getting up early and driving away from the hustle and bustle of Ghana's capital, it felt as though we had entered a scene from the Robert De Niro and Jeremy Irons film, *The Mission*. It was three years since my trip to Uganda; I was now on my medical elective at the University of Ghana's Teaching Hospital, and on this Saturday, I was taking a trip with my adopted church.

To a British suburbanite, I had finally reached "real" Africa. Sure, my first three months in Ghana's capital, Accra, were very different from anything I had experienced in pretty Middle England where I grew up—J.R.R. Tolkien's inspiration for Hobbiton and the Shire—but Accra was still a city. This was something else.

A clearing in the jungle had long ago made way for a village of thatched-roofed circular wooden huts. Electricity and all the modern conveniences that go with it were still to come to this village. There could have been, perhaps, a battery-operated radio, but little else.

We had come at the request of the village chief to run a small health clinic, which mainly consisted of checking people's blood pressures. After we had given out health advice on preventing heart disease and hypertension and distributed a few different medicines, we gave a talk on another hidden illness similar to high blood pressure but also quite different, a deeper sickness that had scoured humanity since the first humans: sin.

Everyone listened patiently, and there was tremendous joy amongst our team as it seemed the entire village stood up in positive response to our plea to surrender their lives to Jesus and come to Him to heal them of this particular sickness. Through the translator, we checked to see if they understood why they were standing, but nobody sat down in response to the clarification. This had been the answer to many prayers from my adopted church, and the work would now only just begin as they sought to disciple those who had responded. But that was for the future.

There was, however, still one more highlight at the end of an amazing day: after the meeting, a mother and a young boy came up to our group and asked for prayer. Her son had stopped talking a few months back and when we asked why, his mother told us that his older brother was training to be a witch doctor and had reported to his younger brother that "he had sold his brother's soul" to advance in his craft.[2]

The mother took the boy to the local hospital to treat his dumbness, but the medics had told her that this was a spiritual problem and they couldn't help. His mother had even taken him to the psychiatric department to see if they could help but had been given the same response. This poor, rural Ghanaian who only knew a life of subsistence farming and bartering with other villagers for daily needs had probably used all the money her family had ever had to reach that district hospital—only to receive such confusing news. The experts there couldn't help. What had she left to hope in?

Through a translator we asked what her son's views on spirituality were, and his mother assured me that both she and her son were Christians and had trusted in Jesus for their salvation. My

2. Christian theology teaches that selling souls is not possible, but lies can still have a powerful effect on us if we allow ourselves to believe them—which is why Jesus declared that it is the *truth* that will set us free.

adopted church had started a church in the village about a year before, and this mother and son were active members. We agreed that it seemed to be a spiritual problem. Despite now knowing Jesus, years of immersion in the culture of witch doctors had obviously created a fear of their power. Whether out of fear or out of a belief that his brother's words acted like a curse, the boy had stopped speaking. We spent a moment telling him the good news that Jesus had authority over fear and the spiritual realm and had the power to change the situation.

Our team prayed a few short prayers with him, declaring truth and asking Jesus to intervene in the situation. After we prayed, he started vocalizing sounds. His mother broke into tears because these were the first sounds he had uttered from his mouth in three months. His voice box had been out of action for so long, one of my senior colleagues assured me it would take a few days for him to form words again, but soon he would be back to normal. Evil had conspired circumstances to make him dumb, but Jesus had a different plan—one of health.

⌒

In contrast to the African tribal boy, Amy had grown up in a middle class, white family in the westernized, hustling city of Johannesburg, South Africa. She was descended from Europeans who had made the dangerous, three-month-long journey by ship many generations ago.

For a couple of years, Amy had had periods of strange illness. She had gone to lots of doctors and been prayed for countless times. Her church friends thought that it must either be spiritual or psychological but this didn't seem to ring true to Amy. Before we married, Michelle had been in the same church as Amy and had invited her over to see if I could make sense of things. For whatever reason, Amy couldn't make the date we set, and somehow we never rescheduled.

A year or so later, Amy was visiting Michelle when I happened to walk in the door. Prompted by the Holy Spirit, I stopped what I was doing, listened to her story, and the various fragments seemed to fall into place. Six weeks previously she had had a scan that revealed the diagnosis but somehow her family doctor hadn't picked this up. Recognizing that her symptoms could all be explained by what was called a multinodular toxic goiter—a condition of the thyroid gland—I urged her to book an appointment with an endocrinologist.

Disillusioned by many trips to specialists that were unfruitful, she was reluctant to try again on yet another doctor's advice—and this one wasn't even practicing medicine but working full time as a pastor! So, in my attempts to persuade her I resorted to that essential modern doctor's handbook: Wikipedia. Through it I showed her how everything fitted together. Her eyes showed a glimmer of hope that this painful two-year journey might have an end. I urged her to go to her family and see if somebody would sponsor the appointment.

Thankfully she was able to go to the appointment, a diagnosis was made, treatment started, and her symptoms all fell away. I saw her again recently, and she said she feels like a completely different person! Somehow, over a couple of years, the enemy had created an environment of confusion and despair, but Jesus, through the guidance of His Spirit, had come to her rescue.

⌣

Hannah and her husband Jim had been attending our church since it first started thirteen years before. When Hannah was twelve years old, she had fallen off a horse and damaged her hip. Since then, for forty-three years, she had been troubled with backache.

During a series on the book of Acts, I spoke on the topic of healing and invited people afterwards to receive prayer. I am not sure why, but Hannah didn't get a chance to be prayed for that week, so she found me the following Sunday and asked if I could pray for her.

My routine in praying for back issues is to sit people down and see if one leg is shorter than the other, because a lot of backaches are caused by slightly different leg lengths. Orthopedic surgeons measure this routinely and distinguish between true leg length discrepancies (when one of the shin or thigh bones is shorter on one leg than the other) and apparent leg length discrepancies (when the shin and thigh bones are the same length, but because of a problem at the hip, the leg is pulled up and appears shorter). After a Sunday service wasn't the appropriate time to get a tape measure out and start measuring points to see if there was a problem at the hip, or if one side hadn't grown as much as the other. However, when Hannah sat square in the chair and I compared her extended legs, it was quite obvious to me, and her accompanying friend, that her left leg looked an inch shorter than her right.

The week before, after my talk on healing, I had prayed for five people with backaches. Three had had one leg shorter than the other and two had had legs the same length. To the joy of everybody around, as we prayed for the people with slightly different leg lengths we saw all three legs grow to equal their counterparts. One of them was a guy in his twenties, named Grant; when we measured his legs, his knees were level but his right ankle was sitting one centimeter shorter than his left. We checked that his hips were square and concluded that his right shin bone was shorter than his left, which he said sounded true because for as long as he could remember he had always worn down the heel of his left shoe more than his right.

We prayed a simple prayer and within a couple of seconds his right leg grew to the same length as his left. There were quite a few people around when we prayed for Grant and we could all see that his knees didn't move and yet his legs were now the same length!

He stood up and said it was weird because he always had felt a little tilted, but for the first time, he now felt level. It took him a week to adjust to walking differently. To this day he has been free of back pain, and now the heels of his shoes wear down evenly.

Hannah had heard about these miracles the week before and that had given her faith to also ask for prayer. As she sat on the chair, with me cross-legged on the floor in front of her cupping her ankles and a few friends gathered around, we prayed for Hannah. Something dramatic happened. Rather than the gentle feeling the others had felt as their leg lengthened, Hannah's whole leg shook violently. All of us were quite shocked, me and Hannah included. As it was happening I watched her hip seem to drop and come forward. When I looked down at her ankles, I saw that they were now level. I asked Hannah to stand, and she started to cry as she realized her legs were straight and the back pain had gone! Wonderfully, her back pain remains healed to this day.

⌇

These short stories may have brought some questions to the surface. How do we process sickness and healing? How do we find God's will in all of it? Why do some get healed instantly, some, like Hannah, live with the sickness for decades before healing happens, and still others die from (or with) their sickness? How does the biblical character of a loving, just God stand up to these seeming inconsistencies?

If you have ever seen anybody paint a watercolor, you'll know that it is important to paint the layers of the background first; then, after the background has dried, one can paint in the details. Similarly, before we hone in on sickness and look at some of the specific, detailed answers to these questions, I want to zoom out and paint the wash, the background, looking at how sickness fits into God's overall redemptive story.

GOD'S HEALTH BIAS

After six years at university I remember very well the day my colleagues and I passed our final exams and transitioned from being a "Mr." to a "Dr." One of the medical insurance firms had got hold of our names in advance and very shrewdly made up smart badges with our new names and titles. I wore my "Dr. Andrew Butterworth" badge with pride as we celebrated and showed it to all my family.

A few years later, the UK had a series of gasoline strikes, which led to a limited fuel supply. At one point all the gas stations were closed except to those who were considered to be doing essential services. Working as a hospital doctor counted as an essential service, so I was able to draw up to the station, show my hospital badge, and fill up. There wasn't anything special about me that got me onto that forecourt apart from my role as a healer, and the title on my badge that backed it up.

Names and titles can mean a lot—as we British should know more than anyone else, with our love for hierarchy and protocol. God's names, too, can mean a lot. There was a time, centuries and millennia ago, recounted in Exodus, chapter 15, when the Israelites had nothing to drink but bitter water, so God showed Moses a certain log to throw into the water to sweeten it. Once the water became drinkable, God made a promise to them, saying that if they chose to obey him, He wouldn't put on them any of the diseases He had put on the Egyptians. And to prove it, He revealed one of His many names to them: *Yahweh Rophe*, "I am the Lord your healer."

It should be unsurprising that one of God's names/titles is Healer because healing and health are His overwhelming bias. Have a look at the reasons for this:

1. He is completely sickness-free.

There is no record of God ever being sick. It is entirely inconsistent with His character. When Jesus walked the earth, even though He touched contagious lepers and many other infectious diseases, He is never mentioned as being sick. Leprosy was so contagious and devastating that lepers were forced to constantly ring a bell to warn people to avoid them, but rather than move away from them, Jesus moved toward them. And rather than the bacteria contaminating Jesus when He made skin-to-skin contact with the lepers, the bacteria chose to flee when it felt His fingers.

2. His home is, always has, and always will be sickness-free.

In the Bible, the name Zion is used poetically to refer to the place where God dwells. In the prophecy of Isaiah, we are told, *"No one living in Zion will say, 'I am ill'"* (Isaiah 33:24 NIV). In John's vision of heaven, a voice confidently declared that in the future heaven, there would no longer be any *"mourning, nor crying, nor pain anymore, for the former things have passed away"* (Revelation 21:4).

3. He created the world sickness-free.

In Genesis chapter 2, God looks at his creation and pronounces it "good," which, in Hebrew terminology, means "made perfect, without blemish." It is only after Adam and Eve sin and are expelled from the garden of Eden that decay and sickness enter the world.

4. When He initiated His kingdom, He made people sickness-free.

"And Jesus went throughout all the cities and villages, teaching in their synagogues and proclaiming the gospel of the kingdom and healing every disease and every affliction" (Matthew 9:35). Amazingly, the gospel accounts show that all those who came to Jesus had their sickness removed. There isn't a single example of someone approaching Jesus and not receiving healing. For example, after Peter had started following Jesus, he invited Jesus to stay at his house and Jesus healed Peter's mother-in-law.[3] A Roman centurion came to Jesus asking Him to heal his servant, and with a word, healing was granted.[4] Jairus, the synagogue ruler, begged Jesus to

3. See Luke 4:39.
4. See Matthew 8:5–13.

heal his daughter and on His way there a woman extracted healing from Jesus by touching His cloak. Once Jesus reached Jairus' house He brought the daughter back to life.[5]

Additionally, all ten of the lepers that approached Jesus for skin cleansing received complete healing, even though only one was thankful.[6] Blind Bartimaeus regained his sight after he ignored the crowd and called out to Jesus for mercy, and at the Pool of Bethesda there were many sick reportedly waiting for an angel to stir the water and yet the man lame for thirty-eight years discovered Jesus and received instant healing.[7] What might have happened if the others discovered Jesus too?

There are twenty-five separate accounts of Jesus bringing physical healing to individuals or groups and exactly zero accounts of sick people being sent away unhealed. In addition, John, His closest disciple, reported this in his gospel account: *"Now there are also many other things that Jesus did. Were every one of them to be written, I suppose that the world itself could not contain the books that would be written"* (John 21:25).

5. When He commissioned His followers, He gave them His authority to heal sickness and give people a foretaste of the future sickness-free kingdom.

On sending out the twelve, the seventy-two, and then all the disciples at His final commissioning, He consistently told them to heal the sick.[8] On commissioning Paul, Jesus instructed Ananias to lay hands on him and cure his blindness.[9] As Paul was healed from his blindness, he was commissioned to go to the Gentiles. During these missionary trips, Paul performed such a number of miraculous healings that the Bible chooses not to list them all, simply saying while on Malta he healed many diseases, and

---

5. See Mark 5:22–43.
6. See Luke 17:12–19.
7. See Mark 10:46–52; John 5:2–9.
8. See Matthew 10:1; Luke 10:1, 2, 9; Mark 16:17–18.
9. See Acts 9:10–12.

during his two-year stay in Ephesus he performed *"extraordinary miracles,"* even remotely, through the use of handkerchiefs and aprons.[10] When the Bible does list healings they are quite dramatic, such as Eutychus' rising from the dead and the healing of the man in Lystra who had been lame from birth.[11] Peter saw similar instances, even the healing of people by his shadow passing over them.[12]

Jesus' commission in the last chapter of Mark states that those who believe will be able to heal the sick, and this is demonstrated in the book of Acts with non-apostles such as Stephen and Philip performing many healing miracles.[13] Supernatural healing is carried on through church history with Christians being used by Jesus to heal many sick and diseased in every century, right through to the present, including well-known church fathers witnessing and carrying out healings such as Augustine of Hippo and Martin Luther (see the Appendix for a list of instances).

6. When He returns to usher in His kingdom, He will make the whole of creation sickness-free.

When I was quite young I had an incredibly vivid dream: in my dream, I looked up to the sky and suddenly Jesus had returned surrounded by a multitude of beings; some people on the earth rose to meet Him in the air while others carried on trying to fix a disintegrating earth. I don't remember much after that but I remember wondering why everybody had not risen to meet Him in the air, because in an instant their bodies were changed and were sickness-free. The apostle Paul describes this future event this way:

> For the Lord himself will descend from heaven with a cry of command, with the voice of an archangel, and with the sound of the trumpet of God. And the dead in Christ will rise first. Then we who are alive, who are left, will be caught up together

---

10. See Acts 28:8–9; 19:11–12.
11. See Acts 20:9–12; 14:8–10.
12. See Acts 5:12–16.
13. See Mark 16:17; Acts 8:6–8, 13.

*with them in the clouds to meet the Lord in the air, and so we
will always be with the Lord.*   (1 Thessalonians 4:16–17)

*For the trumpet will sound, the dead shall be raised imperish-
able, and we shall be changed. For the perishable must clothe itself
with the imperishable, and the mortal with immortality.*
(1 Corinthians 15:52–53 NIV)

Our bodies perish because of decay or sickness, but when we
receive imperishable bodies at Jesus' return, then sickness cannot
affect us. Paul gives another metaphor earlier in the passage: *"So
is it with the resurrection of the dead. What is sown is imperishable;
what is raised is imperishable…It is sown in weakness; it is raised in
power"* (1 Corinthians 15:42–43).

This current body is like a seed that is sown into the ground;
once the plant shoots up, the seed fades from view. Whether the seed
has some marks or imperfections is long forgotten because everyone
only sees the glory of the flower. For those of us who are believers, so
it will be with our new bodies. When God ushers in His kingdom,
the imperfection of the old body will hardly be a consideration. In
Revelation, we see the promise that city of God will come down to
earth and God will dwell with us permanently. All pain, crying, and
death disappear. Sickness will be no more and creation will be set
free as we live in the joy of our resurrection bodies.[14]

KEY POINTS:

1. Sickness brings us into intense vulnerability.

2. God shows no partiality—He will personally engage
   with us and our heartfelt questions, regardless of who
   we are or what our situation.

3. One of God's titles is Healer (*Yahweh Rophe*) because
   His bias is always toward our health.

14. See Revelation 21:2, 4; Romans 8:21.

CHAPTER 2:

SEEING THE BIG PICTURE

"Sickness is mankind's greatest defect."
—*Georg C. Lichtenberg*
Eighteenth-century German scientist

SICKNESS'S DARK BACKSTORY[15]

Picture a place of perfection. A place where everything works and nothing decays; at its helm, the most perfect, benevolent government the universe has ever known. Why would somebody want to upset a place like this—let alone attempt a coup? But that's what happened. No, I am not talking about the fall in the garden of Eden. I am talking about something that happened much earlier.

We aren't given much detail about it, but we know that a very high-ranking angel called Lucifer led a rebellion against God.[16]

15. Much of the theology in this chapter has been developed from a talk by PJ Smyth entitled "Suffering, Sickness, and Healing" given at the Together on a Mission conference in Brighton, UK, on 14 July 2011.
16. See Isaiah 14:12–14; Ezekiel 28:12–18 alludes to it; and Revelation 12 describes it apocalyptically.

Seemingly unhappy with his position in creation, Lucifer set himself up as a rival god to the Father Almighty. But as a created being, it was rather like an ant deciding to set himself up as an alternative president of the United States. Jesus was present when it happened, recounting that He saw Satan *"fall like lightning from heaven"* (Luke 10:18). With him went a third of God's angels, and, no longer looking very angelic, from this point forward they were referred to as demons or devils.[17]

Before his fall, Lucifer would have been an eternally beautiful being, but because of his lust for power and total indulgence in pride, he has distorted into the ugly, snarling, sneering enemy of God. Consumed by hatred, he hates everything about God. If there is any being in the universe whose emotion toward us could be the opposite of God, it is Satan. To get a sense of his character, just look at the names the Bible uses for him: the devil, dragon, serpent, enemy, tempter, murderer, Father of Lies, adversary, accuser, destroyer, and, just simply, the evil one.

When God created humans, Lucifer saw his chance. He and his fellow fallen angels chose to adopt the plot line of many a movie since—unable to hurt the Hero (God) they went after the ones He loved (us). As we are beings created in God's image, Satan was determined to do everything he could to distort that image. The accuser (literally, "Satan") lied to us, telling us that God was unjust and unloving, and tempted us to seize power and all its illicit benefits for ourselves. Tragically, it was a sham—and we humans traded something authentic and precious for a counterfeit, cutting ourselves off from God.

You may have heard the popular biblical phrase that you reap what you sow.[18] Through that act of disobedience, we humans reaped a judgment by God of death.[19] That day, a new entity came into the universe: mortality. Unlike the beings in heaven, our

17. See Revelation 12:3–9.
18. See Galatians 6:7.
19. See Genesis 2:16–17.

physical bodies became subject to decay, and decay leads only to death.

The tragedy was that this was never meant to be. Jesus' human body didn't decay.[20] Heavenly angels don't decay. And as beings made in Jesus' image we weren't meant to decay. It was never the intention of God for creation to experience decay, but because of our rebellion decay happened.

THE PROBLEM OF DECAY

The letter to the Roman church tells us that not only do our bodies become subject to decay but, as stewards of the earth, our rebellion caused the whole of creation to experience decay. Paul informs us that it is not just Jesus' followers who are longing for His return, but that there is a deeper groan that comes from creation as it, too, lives under this slavery.[21]

Just as tooth decay has the capacity to corrupt the whole tooth if left untreated, so, too, does creation decay have an equal pervasiveness. Creation decay affects everything. It is the reason there isn't balance in the world and why natural disasters happen. Its scope is from the macro to the micro; it both causes earthquakes and corrupts the DNA of viruses and bacteria to make them disease-causing.

Would you believe me if I told you there are actually more cells of "good" bacteria living inside us than cells that "belong" to our body? Because of their much smaller size, if bacteria could vote against the cells of our body they would win hands down by sheer numbers. Before you recoil from thinking about a body full of bacteria, it is sobering to note that without these helpful bacteria we'd soon cease to function. They do millions of essential processes for us every second, without which we'd die. Bacteria have a bad name

20. See Acts 2:31.
21. See Romans 8:21–22.

now, but that's just because creation decay messed some of them up; they were created to be good.

Viruses are in a similar boat. Unlike bacteria, they are not even living creatures—just bits of DNA floating in casing that has been borrowed from a host. However, only 1 percent of all viruses cause disease. The rest carry out their original job of maintaining balance in our ecosystem. In Genesis 1, when God declared everything created as "good," He meant even viruses and bacteria.

Decay, however, brought chaos, and chaos, unlike God, isn't fair in how it distributes itself. Like a whirlwind that wreaks havoc quite randomly, or the injuries that occur through the spray of bullets in a battle scene, from our perspective on earth there is not fairness to how we get affected by creation decay. For example:

+ Because of decay, some people are born with a full set of limbs, but others are not.

+ Because of decay, some people are born with cancers already developing inside them or with the genetic time bomb of a cancer developing later in life. But the other two thirds of the population will never develop any form of cancer.[22]

+ Because of decay, some of us will be affected by one or more of the seven hundred or so distinct genetically-caused diseases or one or more of the many more diseases that have a genetic influence—but others will not.[23]

The bullets of genetic decay are not discerning in their choice. Like rain, they fall on both the righteous and the unrighteous, and specific bullets, to the puzzlement of many a psalmist and philosopher, may hit the righteous but miss the wicked.[24] Take, for instance, the man born blind who was brought to Jesus. *"And his*

22. Cancer Research UK, "Lifetime Risk of Cancer," http://www. cancerresearchuk.org/cancer-info/cancerstats/incidence/risk/ (accessed 15 May 2015).
23. "List of genetic disorders," Wikipedia, http://en.wikipedia.org/wiki/List_of_ genetic_disorders (accessed 15 May 2015).
24. See Matthew 5:44–45.

disciples asked him, 'Rabbi, who sinned, this man or his parents, that he was born blind?' Jesus answered, 'It was not that this man sinned, or his parents'" (John 9:2–3). Neither he nor his parents had caused his blindness. The fall of man caused it by ushering in decay. Think of all the problems in the world today, and you can trace each one back to the fall of man and its precedent, the fall of angels. So, shouldn't our anger be directed there?

Well, it is right to be angry at the destruction that Satan and his demons have sown, and continue to sow, but we shouldn't make the mistake of putting the rest of it on Adam and Eve. Every one of us did our part in tainting God's perfect world with our rebellion and selfish ways. If sin brought in decay, aren't all of us responsible? R. C. Sproul puts it this way:

> Sin is cosmic treason. Sin is treason against a perfectly pure Sovereign. It is an act of supreme ingratitude toward the One to whom we owe everything, to the One who has given us life itself. Have you ever considered the deeper implications of the slightest sin, of the minutest peccadillo? What are we saying to our Creator when we disobey Him at the slightest point? We are saying no to the righteousness of God. We are saying, "God, Your law is not good. My judgment is better than Yours. Your authority does not apply to me. I am above and beyond Your jurisdiction. I have the right to do what I want to do, not what You command me to do.[25]

In 1910, the author G. K. Chesterton published a book entitled *What's Wrong with the World*. The story goes that the book came about because, two years earlier, *The Times* (London) had asked a number of authors to submit essays around that same question. Fed up with the blame-shifting and the finger-pointing of the other essayists, G. K. turned the debate inward by submitting the following response:

---

25. R. C. Sproul, *The Holiness of God* (Carol Stream, IL: Tyndale, 2000, 2nd ed.), 116.

Dear Sirs,

I am.

Sincerely yours,

G. K. Chesterton

Who is at fault for sickness in the world? Dear Sirs, I am. Sincerely yours, [insert your own name here]. It was we who opened Pandora's Box. God's heart wasn't for sickness to enter the world, but in our rebellion we caused it. That's right—we— you and I. Not just Adam, not just Hitler, not just your next-door neighbor. Sickness is here because of *us*.

If we are blaming God, or putting all our anger on Adam and Eve or the devil, then we are in danger because the road to healing starts by admitting our part of the problem, no matter how innocent we feel, or how uninvolved we were with our current sickness coming to us. Ultimately, sickness is here because of sin, and not one of us is innocent of sin.

SICKNESS ON THE TIMELINE OF GOD

But if God is all-powerful, why doesn't He put an end to sickness? If we look at the timeline of God, the short answer to that question is—He will! From God's perspective, sickness, like sin, while extremely significant to us, will only be present in the universe for an extremely short time—nestled on either side of eternity.

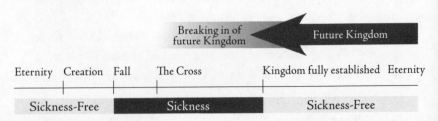

Sickness came in through the fall but is eradicated when Jesus' kingdom is fully established. On either side of these events is eternity. However, for those of us affected by sickness, this short period where sickness is present is still extremely significant.

Before we look at how to process this, I think it's important to put our experience of sickness in the context of the Christian's great hope: If we have become one of God's children, then He guarantees that He will remove sickness from us for all eternity. The American evangelist D. L. Moody spoke of it this way:

> Some day you will read in the papers that D. L. Moody of East Northfield, is dead. Don't you believe a word of it! At that moment I shall be more alive than I am now; I shall have gone up higher, that is all, out of this old clay tenement into a house that is immortal—a body that death cannot touch, that sin cannot taint; a body fashioned like unto His glorious body.

"A body fashioned like unto His glorious body" is a hope indeed—especially for those who are suffering in their body through sickness. Even if our body dies contorted by sickness or riddled with cancer, if Jesus has regenerated us spiritually then we will have a fully healed new body for the rest of eternity. David Fairchild, senior pastor of Trinity West Seattle writes:

> *"For if we have been united with him in a death like his, we shall certainly be united with him in a resurrection like his"* (Romans 6:5). As my wife, Grace, and I sat on either side of her passing mother, Connie, we felt strangely and happily awkward for having so much hope, as if we had a secret just between us. There was a moment Grace and I made eye contact and a wry smile crept across my wife's lips. Were we supposed to feel this way? Was it wrong to feel so joyful in such a difficult situation?

We loved Connie dearly. This was a beautiful and hard-working Latina woman who grew up without the material comforts most enjoy in Southern California. She was as physically strong as she was personally shy. But in the last two years, her cancer physically broke her. And through the deterioration of her body, the Lord answered our prayers and brought her to a living faith in the living Christ. She spent the last year and a half bringing her family members with her to church to hear the gospel until her body denied her mobility. And when the doctors gave the heart-breaking news that her cancer had spread and chemotherapy was no longer an option, she warmly said, "I guess I get to meet my Savior even sooner!"

We miss Connie. But we will not miss her forever.

Connie's cancer was not wasted. She knew her frail, hollowed husk was not permanent and would one day be traded for a resurrection body—a body just like her Savior's. She held hope to her heart like a warm drink on a cold day. She was convinced that her death was an end to her suffering sighs and struggle with sin. And through Jesus' death her life was about to begin. In her last few breaths, I had the honor of whispering this revealed mystery to her, reminding her of what, in only a moment, she would know far better than I.

We miss Connie. But we will not miss her forever. Praise to the One who puts death to death![26]

Like the examples given in the previous chapter, as God's kingdom breaks in, some of us may experience healing here on earth. Others of us may be like Connie and only access that healing after our body passes away. But God's promise to His children is that all of us will be fully healed—it's just a question of timing.

---

26. David Fairchild, "A Resurrection Like His,", http://marshill. com/2012/06/23/a-resurrection-like-his (article no longer available).

That may be our future, but how do we understand our sickness now? If sickness came in to the universe through mankind's sin, is our job just to wait it out? Not at all! As we will see in later chapters, there is a lot we can do to respond to sickness, but first we must understand sickness as being part of a dynamic process that we can significantly influence.

Four main influencers affect this dynamic: ourselves, other humans, Satan and demons, and God. While it may be tempting to view these on equal footing, because God is the Creator, and Satan, demons and human beings are all created beings, this means that God is able to stand above these other influencers on sickness and restrict and limit sickness, as we will explore further in chapter 4.

THE FOUR INFLUENCERS ON SICKNESS

OURSELVES

As well as being responsible for ushering sickness into the world, we humans have a large responsibility for the high levels of sickness we experience because of the everyday choices we make. For example, on many occasions I have pushed myself leading up to a holiday, only to get there and find that my body collapses and seems to invite in all the bacteria and viruses in the surrounding neighborhood to come and invade.

For more serious illnesses, such as cancer, the lead-time is far longer. Take, for instance, the teenage girl who starts smoking one or two cigarettes on weekends. In her twenties, she's the career woman who relies on cigarettes as much as coffee to give her a pick-up when she is on edge or stressed out; by her thirties, she has developed a life-long forty-a-day habit. If her genes are like the majority of the population, once she reaches sixty years, her chances of dying from lung cancer are one in thirty-five—and, let me stress, that refers to people who die from, not just contract, lung cancer.[27] Forty-five years or so after she made that initial decision to give a cigarette a try, she will likely be looking at a diagnosis of lung cancer. With these sorts of scenarios, there is often a sense of regret and/or injustice that circumstances forced illness upon us, but at a deeper level there is often a knowledge that we played a part in our fate.

Science has recently shown that our choices are much more deeply intertwined with our health than we may have realized, and in the next chapter we'll look at how what we think dramatically shapes our physiology, and specifically, our immune system's ability to resist sickness in quite dramatic ways.

OUR FELLOW HUMAN BEINGS

The seventeenth-century British poet John Donne famously wrote that no man is an island. If you have you ever caught the flu by sitting next to somebody on a crowded bus or plane, you'll be able to relate to that statement. And what if there were a chance that you would catch something far more serious than the standard influenza?

On February 21, 2003, Liu Jianlun, a sixty-four-year-old doctor from the Guangdong province of China, was showing symptoms of a fever. Despite not feeling well, he chose to keep his flight to Hong Kong in order to make it to a family wedding. In doing so, he infected six other guests with his illness at the hotel where he was staying.

One of the six, an American businessman, Johnny Chen, took a flight to Hanoi, Vietnam, and there began to develop symptoms of a fever, headache, dry cough and some breathing difficulties. He was admitted to a local hospital, The French Hospital of Hanoi, with what was thought to be a bad case of the flu. There,

27. See http://nomograms.mskcc.org/Lung/Screening.aspx. Based on an average of five cigarettes per day for five years, twenty cigarettes per day for ten years, and forty cigarettes per day for thirty years.

his mystery illness quickly infected twenty health care workers, including noted Italian epidemiologist Carlo Urbani, who worked at the Hanoi World Health Organization (WHO) office.

Dr. Urbani had provided medical care for Mr. Chen and realized that it wasn't the flu that was giving him his symptoms, but something far worse. He quickly notified WHO and a rapid response was started that is credited with vastly reducing the extent of the outbreak.[28] On February 28, 2003, Dr. Urbani realized he had discovered a new disease, which he named Severe Acute Respiratory Syndrome (SARS).

Less than two weeks after making the discovery of SARS, Dr. Urbani flew to speak at a conference in Bangkok but felt feverish on the plane. He was immediately taken to a hospital and placed in isolation. His wife was able to talk to him via an intercom and she saw him conscious only once before he was put on a respirator. After eighteen days of intensive care, at the age of forty-six, and leaving behind three children, Dr. Urbani passed away.

SARS turned out to be a very potent infection, spreading from Hong Kong to thirty-seven countries and infecting eight thousand people. Approximately 10 percent of those who were infected died—from all stages and walks of life. Sadly, Liu Jianlun, Johnny Chen, and Dr. Urbani were among those fatalities.

From the benefit of hindsight, it is easy to ponder what would have happened if Liu Jianlun had decided not to go to the wedding in Hong Kong. Would Dr. Urbani's children still have had their father with them? Would the relatives of the other eight hundred fatalities still have their loved ones with them? We may never know the answers to those specific questions, but what is quite clear is that the SARS outbreak had been growing in the Guangdong Province of China for several months prior to February 2002. If

28. Global Alert and Response, "Dr. Carlo Urbani of the World Health Organization Dies of SARS," World Health Organization, March 29, 2003, http://www.who.int/csr/sars/urbani/en/ (accessed 15 May 2015).

not Mr. Jianlun, it would have been somebody else who carried SARS out of China and triggered so many cases round the world.

How do you respond, however, when sickness has been brought entirely through somebody else's actions, like the child I saw back in my hospital days who'd had numerous bones broken through the actions of an aggressive, angry, ill-coping parent—actions that affected that child for the rest of his life? Or the wife I met who had become HIV positive through her husband's sexual infidelity? Not only did she have to process what this meant for her marriage, but she also had to come to terms with taking three potent antivirals, with quite serious side-effects, for the rest of her life—each pill acting as a reminder of his costly mistake and betrayal.

Or what about the numerous babies I saw born to intravenous drug-addicted mothers who started to go through "cold turkey" withdrawal the day they were born? If they were worse off, they may also have been infected with Hepatitis C, with a small proportion of them going through childhood with their livers slowly turning to scar tissue, leading to liver failure or liver cancer in adult life. My eyes start to water as I think back to those little babies I briefly cared for in the special care baby unit and how their lives may have turned out today.

We can't even imagine the countless millions of people who have been victims to diseases that have flourished because of squalid man-made living conditions. As part of my time in Ghana, I visited the fifteenth-century Elmina Castle, the oldest European building in existence below the Sahara. Here, thousands upon thousands of captured Africans were held until they could be boarded onto ships to be sold to plantation owners in the New World. As we walked around what can only be described as a dungeon, the guide told us that people would be so cramped, they could barely stand or move while they waited to board a ship. The slaves would defecate in buckets that would often stay in the room for days at a time. Infectious diseases such as cholera or dysentery claimed the lives of whole families.

After seeing the living quarters for slaves I thought the worst was over, but upstairs we found a very different room that, in a way, was even more horrendous. It was a chapel. As I looked around the simply decorated church building with its wooden pews and pulpit, I pictured eighteenth-century Europeans singing songs like "All Creatures of Our God and King" or preaching about God's love for humanity, while in the floor below they had enslaved and locked away their fellow creation, treating them worse than animals and making them sick from disease.

We may not have been slave traders, but, whoever we are and wherever we are, by putting our needs ahead of others', we have all contributed in some way to the quantity of sickness in the world today.

SATAN AND HIS DEMONS

Satan loves sickness. It is a weapon he will try to wield at every opportunity to bring harm to humanity. Jesus told us that Satan's aim is to *"steal and kill and destroy"* (John 10:10), and sickness is commonly one of his favored means. Specifically, Satan is named in bringing about a spinal disfigurement in a woman who Jesus healed and approximately 25 percent of Jesus' healings in the gospel of Mark involve demons in the direct cause of the disease.[29] In Peter's first sermon to Gentile believers, he said about Jesus, *"He went about doing good and healing all who were oppressed by the devil"* (Acts 10:38).

I have told you already about the boy who went dumb in response to his brother's occult involvement, but there was another occasion in Ghana when I met a person at a prayer meeting whose witch doctor relative had cast a spell against him, and he'd developed what seemed like pharyngeal candidiasis (a yeast infection

---

29. See Luke 13:16.

of the lower throat), that, after prayer, went away as quickly as it came.

In the parts of the world where witchcraft and occultism are common, overt, demonically instigated disease is well known. In the rest of the world, however, the link to sickness is less direct—but still very significant. With a third of all the created angels under his control, Satan deploys them in an unseen battle for our will. Suggestions are made, truth is distorted, and sin is glorified. "You can drive home; you've done it before" might be a temptation that, if followed by the drunk driver, may lead to an innocent passerby being confined to a wheelchair. Satan is elated, because God's image is distorted and a chance is created to whisper to the victim, "See? God doesn't care—He can't even stop a drunk driver from crippling you. He must really hate you to abandon you like that!" Satan uses sickness to try and drive a wedge between God and us, but in doing so he is true to his name—the Father of Lies. Any idea that God wishes harm for us is just that—a lie from the Father of Lies.

To illustrate, I'll take us back to the story of Job: "*So Satan went out from the presence of the* Lord *and struck Job with loathsome sores from the sole of his foot to the crown of his head. And he [Job] took a piece of broken pottery with which to scrape himself while he sat in the ashes*" (Job 2:7–8). Satan caused Job's sickness, but he didn't stop there. He went on to discredit God's character and cause Job to blame God for his own handiwork.[30] Once that has happened, it is a simple step for Job to cut off relationship, saying to God: "*Your hands fashioned and made me, and now you have destroyed me altogether... Are not my days few? Then cease, and leave me alone, that I may find a little cheer before I go*" (Job 10:8, 20–21). This is Satan's great propaganda campaign. He uses sickness to tell his great lies: "God desires for you to be like this. God doesn't care. God has abandoned you."

---

30. See Job 3:23.

Lies are powerful things, particularly if they are told to you regularly. Joseph Goebbels, Adolf Hitler's chief of propaganda in Nazi Germany, once said, "If you tell a lie, tell a big one and tell it often." By repeatedly telling the lie that the Jews were the cause of Germany's woes, the Nazi party convinced a nation to vote Nazism into power. People didn't believe it at first, but after relentless campaigning, some started to be convinced. Once in power, the Nazis seized all communication and kept the lie pounding into people's ears and popping up in front of their eyes for years, with a powerful but devastating effect.

Reading the story of Job is similar to watching a gripping movie or seeing a play. The drama of watching a movie often occurs when the characters get duped by the villain into believing that the hero isn't really a hero. We, the watchers, can see the whole thing clearly but for those characters caught in the middle of it, it is not so clear—that is, until the end draws near, and the true natures of the hero and villain are revealed.

It was the same with Job. In the midst of it all, he sees God as the villain, but as the narrative draws to an end God brings him clarity: "*I know that you can do all things...I have uttered what I did not understand...and you make it known to me*" (Job 42:2–4).

And so, foiling Satan's plan, God draws Job far closer to Himself than Job had ever known before, and the result is great blessing: "*I had heard of you...but now my eye sees you*" (Job 42:5). "*And the Lord blessed the latter days of Job more than his beginning.... And Job died, an old man, and full of days*" (Job 42:12, 17).

In God's great story of redemption the end is drawing near; Satan's time of duping believers will soon cease. Against a backdrop of sickness-fueled lies that God isn't good, that God doesn't care, that God isn't fair, a Hero has arrived who has shown us the true character of God: Jesus.

As we said in the opening chapter, God is overwhelmingly anti-sickness and pro-healing. After all, Jesus died to reverse all the effects of sin, including the effect of sickness. All healing, whether here on earth or our full healing in heaven, is accessed through Jesus. However, the Bible does show that, at times, God uses sickness to fulfill His own purposes.

GOD

If you've read the narrative of Moses' life, you'll remember the time God spoke to him out of a bush that had caught fire but strangely wasn't being consumed. At one point, God says, *"Who gave man his mouth? **Who makes him deaf or mute?** Who gives him sight or **makes him blind? Is it not I, the LORD?"** (Exodus 4:11 NIV). Because we have already seen how pro-health and anti-sickness God is, this seems a difficult statement to understand. But it isn't an isolated incident.

In Exodus we read that when the Egyptian nation resisted God's request to release His people from slavery, two (or possibly three) of the ten plagues God sent against them were sickness-related: the boils, the plague on the livestock, and possibly the deaths of all first-borns.[31] In response to the Philistines' capture of the ark of the covenant, God sent cancers on those Philistines nearby.[32] But it wasn't just Israel's enemies on whom God brought sickness. The book of Numbers details how God sent poisonous snakes amongst the Israelites because of their impatience, and that *"many"* (Numbers 21:6) died from being bitten. Then later in the book of Deuteronomy, as well as declaring many blessings for following His commands, God also threatened punishment for not following them, which included various sicknesses:

> *The LORD will strike you with wasting disease and with fever, inflammation and fiery heat,...with the boils of Egypt, and with tumors and scabs and itch...with madness and blindness and confusion of mind...sicknesses grievous and lasting....*

---

31. See Exodus 7–11.
32. See 1 Samuel 5:6.

Every sickness also and every affliction that is not recorded in
the book of this law, the LORD will bring upon you until you,
are destroyed.   (Deuteronomy 28:22, 27, 28, 59, 61)

Much later on, because of King Jehoram's evil practices, God
brought what appears to be terminal bowel cancer on him and
then bubonic plague on his people.[33]

To those of us from a Western mind-set, this may seem difficult to fathom. Would God seriously send sickness? But the Bible
is unapologetic—He does. Like everything in the universe, sickness is available to God to be used by Him for His purposes. You
may recall that God used foreign nations to bring judgment on
Judah and Israel; using sickness doesn't seem any different—and
certainly King David, at least, considered it kinder. When David
disobeyed God and took a census to massage his own ego, God
offered him three options as consequences.[34] David chose three
days of God-sent sickness over three months of enemy attack or
three years of famine because he argued that God's mercy is far
greater than being placed in the hands of humans.

These are all examples from the Old Testament. In the New
Testament, God's character doesn't change; He still uses sickness
in judgment, but now, through the death and resurrection of Jesus,
we have protection from that judgment.

For example, God used Paul to supernaturally place blindness
on the sorcerer Elymas, whose dark arts were being used to dis-
courage the island's governor from hearing the gospel.[35] And as
an unbeliever, Paul himself was blinded by Jesus on the Damascus
Road.[36] In what seems to be parallel to the judgment plagues in
Egypt, the book of Revelation shows there will be three sets of

---

33. See http://www.ncbi.nlm.nih.gov/pubmed/15785440 (accessed 15 May 2015);
2 Chronicles 21:14–15, 19.
34. See 2 Samuel 24:10; 1 Chronicles 21:1–18.
35. See Acts 13:6–12.
36. See Acts 9:8.

seven judgments placed on unbelievers.[37] Sickness is a part of each set of judgments, and God specifically directs the angels to bring these sicknesses on the earth.

In the "seal" judgments, the fourth seal releases two riders of pale horses that are given authority to inflict a quarter of the earth with pestilence (sickness), among other things.[38] In the "trumpet" judgments, the blowing of the third trumpet causes an angel to release something that turns the water bitter. The poisoned water is deadly for some people.[39] Finally, in the "bowl" judgments, the first bowl is poured out by an angel that releases something on to the earth that causes people to develop sores on their skin.[40]

This seems to be a gigantic amount of God-sent sickness. How do we process this? Is this a parallel to the destruction of Jerusalem prior to the city's restoration? Is sickness sent one last time before the world is made sickness-free? Some people take the view that this represents the sicknesses and disasters that humanity has experienced throughout the centuries since Revelation was penned. Others feel it relates to a future event. Either way, God clearly sends sickness. But does He send it on Christian believers?

Perhaps, but never as punishment. The Bible is clear that things are very different for those who worship God *after* Jesus' death and resurrection than for those who worshipped God prior to it. Before the cross, God's people often reaped a judgment of sickness through their actions, but for those of us alive after Jesus' first coming, we know that Jesus has borne our judgment. He *"took our illnesses"* (Matthew 8:17) and became a curse on our behalf.[41] For those of us who trust in Jesus, God's judgment through the use of sickness has been spent.

---

37. Some theologians argue that the judgments are already happening, spread through the centuries. Either way, the point I am making still holds: God seems to be initiating sickness.
38. See Revelation 6:8.
39. See Revelation 8:10–11.
40. See Revelation 16:2.
41. See Galatians 3:13.

So, if there is a final judgment of sickness coming, it is more important than ever that people turn to Jesus because He will be their only protection. Even during the Egyptian judgments when God sent the twelve plagues, it was quite clear that the Israelites were uniquely protected.[42] How much more will those be protected during any final judgment who have already turned to Christ for their salvation, and have been adopted into God's family?

HOW DO WE MAKE SENSE OF THIS?

While it is clear that God has used, and will use, sickness as part of His judgment, Jesus bore the judgment for the sins of those who have repented and been adopted into His family. For example, when Israel repented for the sin that caused God to send the poisonous snakes, God provided a place of healing and foreshadowed the healing that Christ would bring. Similarly, when David repented, God also stopped the judgment process. And, in the New Testament, although God judged Paul with blindness, after Paul showed humility and repentance, God healed him.

Cleansing from sin (and any resultant sickness) follows repentance. When we become believers, we repent of the sin that separates us from God and then receive the guarantee of a future sin-free and sickness-free existence.

As we go on to live lives as believers we continue to repent of sin that we become convicted of, therefore allowing God to bring cleansing to our bodies and halt, or even reverse, any effects the sin may have had within us.[43] The Reformer, Martin Luther, famously wrote in the first of his Ninety-Five Theses: "When our Lord and Master Jesus Christ said 'Repent,' he intended that the entire life of believers should be repentance."[44]

---

42. See Exodus 8:22–23; 9:4, 7, 26; 11:4–7.
43. See 1 John 1:9.
44. Quoted in David Mathis, "Luther's First Thesis and Last Words," DesiringGod.com, October 31, 2008, http://www.desiringgod.org/blog/posts/luthers-first-thesis-and-last-words (accessed 15 May 2015).

As we will see in the next chapter, if we take for granted what Jesus did for us and live in in longstanding, unrepentant rebellion and idolatry, God still reserves the right to use sickness to bring believers to repentance.[45] I don't believe God does this lightly. Instead, He is weighing up the effect of the sickness against the greater harm that unrepentant sin causes. His motive in this is love. It may be similar to a desperate father who might instigate a police charge against his teenage son who repeatedly and willfully takes his car for drunken joy rides. This is not what normal fathers do, but this is not a normal situation. Likewise, it is not Yahweh Rophe's nature to bring sickness except out of a desire to lovingly bring us back to repentance and right relationship.

DRAWING IT ALL TOGETHER

So, to come back to the question at the beginning of the chapter, why would God allow a man to be born blind? Was it caused by his sin or his parents' sin? In His typical fashion, Jesus didn't answer the question directly: Jesus could have stopped and done a teaching session, breaking their personal sin paradigm, but instead He chose the deeper answer. This came about, Jesus explained, *"That the works of God might be displayed in him"* (John 9:3).

You may have the same question of God, and I suspect Jesus will respond in the same way, moving you away from what's happened to what He wants to do. "Why am I sick, God?" "So that I can work it for good—using it as a means to connect deeper with you," He will answer. The big question is: Are you prepared to let Him do this, to work your sickness 'round for your good? I can't promise supernatural healing, but I can promise that if you, like Job, choose to engage with God, He will draw close and engage with you in mercy and love. Perhaps you will take up His offer of eternal healing (if you haven't already) and perhaps He may even demonstrate that future healing power to you here on earth.

---

45. See 1 Corinthians 11:27–32.

Before mankind's sin and disobedience against God, sickness was unknown in the universe. Sickness was ushered in to our world because of us. This situation isn't a static one, but it is affected by four influencers of sickness today: ourselves, our fellow humans, Satan and demons, and God. We have seen from the previous chapter that God allows this situation only temporarily and has made a way to remove sickness from the universe in the future. In chapter 4 we'll look at how we can process this situation for ourselves, but first we look at greater detail at how our own thought processes and perspective on sickness can influence the way we experience sickness.

KEY POINTS:

1. God never intended for His creation to experience decay, but through our rebellion, decay and sickness entered the world.

2. Our current experience of sickness is affected by four factors: ourselves, our fellow human beings, evil, and God.

3. Sickness is only temporary, and God has made a plan to restore His creation to be free of sickness.

CHAPTER 3:

DEFEATING KILLER THOUGHTS

"Medicine, to produce health, must examine disease; and
music, to create harmony, must investigate discord."
—*Plutarch*
First century Greek philosopher

In 1982, Serbian immigrants Duška and Boris Vujicic gave birth
to their son, Nick, in Melbourne, Australia. Duška had had three
normal antenatal scans, but at the birth she and her husband discovered that their son had a very rare condition called tetra-amelia
syndrome, which meant he was missing both arms and both legs.
He had just two small feet, one of which had two toes, attached
directly to his torso.

Nick learned to cope with his condition and attended a
mainstream school, but he was the subject of severe bullying
and, at the age of eight, he became severely depressed. When
he was ten, the ridicule and the sense of being a burden over-
whelmed him, and he unsuccessfully attempted to drown himself in the bath.

Nick's parents were Christians and encouraged him endlessly during this time. He made it through the depression and became a Christian himself:

> [At] age fifteen I gave my life to Jesus after reading John 9. I knew I had to make my life right with Him but I blamed Him for my pain. I read how Jesus said that the blind man was born that way so that the works of God would be revealed through him. I said to God that if He had a plan for that man I certainly believed that He had one for me. I totally surrendered the "needing to know the plan" idea and trusted in Him one day at a time.[46]

He then prayed that God would give him arms and legs. Initially he told God that if his prayer remained unanswered, he would stop praising Him indefinitely. However, a key turning point in his faith came when his mother showed him a newspaper article about a man dealing with a severe disability. Nick realized he was not unique in his struggles and began to embrace his lack of limbs. After this he realized that his accomplishments could inspire others and he became grateful for his life.

Nick gradually figured out how to live a full life without limbs, adapting to many of the daily skills limbed people accomplish without thinking. He writes with the two toes on his left foot and a special grip that slides onto his big toe. He knows how to use a computer and can type up to forty-three words per minute. During his teenage years he taught himself to dress, wash, shave, and even to comb his hair and brush his teeth. He has since gone on to more demanding tasks, such as playing golf, soccer, and sky-diving. He's an author, musician, actor, and his hobbies include fishing, painting, and swimming.

Completing a degree in accounting and financial planning, Nick was intending to follow his father and become an accountant.

---

46. Nick Vujicic, "Bio," Life Without Limbs, http://www.lifewithoutlimbs.org/about-nick (accessed 15 May 2015).

However, from the age of seventeen he had started speaking at Christian prayer groups and saw the hope he could bring to people. At the age of nineteen he set up his own foundation and now gives motivational talks in corporations, colleges, and churches, and has addressed over three million people in over twenty-four countries.

At one point, Nick wondered if he would ever get married, thinking no one would be able to love him. On February 12, 2012, however, Nick married his fiancée, Kanae Miyahara, and a year later she gave birth to their son, Kiyoshi James. Nick's life has changed dramatically. He no longer has the anger he had toward God, and he looks for any opportunity to talk about the transformation Jesus Christ brought about in his life. While he has achieved so much, he still has the hope that one day God may supernaturally heal him, and so he keeps a pair of shoes in his closet just in case.

THE COMMUNICATION BETWEEN THE MIND AND THE IMMUNE SYSTEM

Our mind is a powerful organ, and, as Nick shows us, how we process our experience with sicknesses can massively affect our day-to-day living. Toxic thoughts surrounding his sickness almost led Nick to bring an early end to his life, but once he allowed God to change his thought patterns, his life took a completely different path—one that he could never have imagined. In recent years, science has demonstrated that our thoughts can not only change our experience of sickness but can actually trigger our body to either resist or succumb to some sicknesses. It is something the Bible has alluded to for a long time: *"A joyful heart is good medicine, but a crushed spirit dries up the bones"* (Proverbs 17:22) and *"A tranquil heart gives life to the flesh, but envy makes the bones rot"* (Proverbs 14:30).

In Psalm 32, David also talks about his bones being affected by his thoughts. In relation to failing to confess sin he said: *"when I kept silent, my bones wasted away"* (Psalm 32:3). These verses warn us that toxic mind-sets such as envy, despair, or unrepentance can directly affect things far away in the body, such as our bones.

Why our bones, you may ask? At the center of our bones is our bone marrow, the jelly-like substance that dogs seem to love. Our bone marrow is continuously producing one of the central features of our immune system: our white blood cells. Healthy bone marrow leads to a healthy immune system. But if, for whatever reason, our immune system is unhealthy, it will not be effective in preventing cancerous cells developing, or stopping foreign pathogens from invading, such as viruses, bacteria, funguses, parasites, etc.

Chaos also ensues when our immune system fails to distinguish between what should be attacked and what shouldn't be. Autoimmune diseases occur when our immune system mistakes our own cells as foreign and attacks them. Allergies, such as hay fever, or allergic reactions to animal hair or dust mites, occur when our immune system thinks that harmless foreign objects, such as pollen or parts of a dead dust mite, are actually dangerous, and launches a huge defense. If anyone has ever experienced or witnessed an anaphylactic attack, where the throat and face swell in response to a severe allergic reaction, you'll know the danger of an overactive immune system that decides to pick on harmless substances, such as peanuts or cat fur.

To have a healthy immune system we need to be neither underactive nor overactive, but in perfect balance. Illustrated in the table below is what results when it becomes unbalanced:

	Underactive Immune System	Overactive Immune System
One's Own Tissue	Cancers Tumors	Autoimmune Diseases
Foreign Substances	Viral Bacterial & Fungal infections	Allergies & Anaphylaxis

Science has now born witness to the truth of the Bible by demonstrating that mental stress, depression, and other negative mind-sets can alter our immune system and take it away from the just-right balancing point in between the two extremes.

For instance, researchers from The Ohio State University studied medical students over a ten-year period and found consistently that during exams, the students' immunity dropped.[47] The stress of exams actually led to fewer natural killer cells, weaker T-cells (that fight off viruses and tumors), and a halt in production of immune-boosting gamma interferon. Mental stress has a direct weakening effect on our ability to fight off disease.

Another study was carried out amongst relatives who cared for people with Alzheimer's disease.[48] Alzheimer's is a very difficult disease to deal with because during its course, relatives watch their loved one slowly lose their ability to think and their awareness of who they are or who their loved ones are. While training to be a doctor, I worked as a nursing assistant at my local hospital and cared for patients who were at the end stage of this disease. It was devastating to see these once-intelligent men and women shouting out random words or banging cups repetitively against tables, lost in confusion. This study looked at the development of mild depression in their relatives, which is all too common. What was surprising from their results was that those who developed depression also dropped their immunity. Not only that, the low levels of immune cells lasted, curiously, for at least eighteen months. Clearly how we think has a much longer effect on our bodies than we may have realized.

The good news is that is that this effect can go the other way as well, and a healthy thought life can boost immunity. Researchers from Yale and Stanford Universities looked at people undergoing

---

47. See American Psychological Association, "Stress Weakens the Immune System," http://www.apa.org/research/action/immune.aspx (accessed 15 May 2015).
48. Ibid.

knee surgery.[49] They found that those who responded best to stress had healthier immune systems, which led to quicker recovery rates, knocking weeks off their recovery time compared to those who responded poorly to stress.

How can our thought lives modulate our immune production at the center of our bones? The brain is such a long way from our leg and arm bones! The answer is through a mixture of nerves and local chemicals. Recently this pathway has been mapped, and it is fascinating.

What happens is this: toxic thought patterns in the brain lead to the production of chemicals called pro-inflammatory cytokines (PICs). These PICs send a signal through the vagus nerves, one of the biggest pairs of nerves in the body, which travel out from the brainstem to almost every organ in the body. The nerves then signal for PICs to be produced in the body, which then communicates chemically with our immune system.

Some researchers looking into these phenomena in rats cut the rats' vagus nerves to see what would happen to this brain-immune system communication.[50] Predictably, because the communication was lost, when stressed or depressed, the rats with the cut vagus nerves retained their normal immune function. However, the rats with intact vagus nerves did not and became ill. This is amazing because it means that cutting a pair of nerves can halt the brain-body immune communication. The researchers also found that this communication went both ways. When the rats got physically sick, those with intact vagus nerves developed a sickness response (being more lethargic, developing a fever, etc.), but those rats with cut vagus nerves carried on as if they were well, even though their bodies were fighting off infection the whole time! Furthermore,

---

49. P. H. Rosenberger, et al., "Surgical Stress-Induced Immune Cell Redistribution Profiles Predict Short-Term and Long-Term Postsurgical Recovery. A Prospective Study," *Journal of Bone and Joint Surgery*, 2009.
50. See http://www.apa.org/monitor/dec01/anewtake.aspx (accessed 29 May 2015).

when the rats were well, if the scientist bypassed the vagus nerves and injected some of the PICs directly into the fluid around the rats' brains, then the rats would develop an illness response to this—even when there was no infection in their body. They felt and acted ill, when in fact they weren't.

Can you imagine how useful it would be to be able to cut off this communication? Imagine if, when you are starting to feel ill, there was some way you could block your vagus nerves and carry on feeling mentally well. Unfortunately it is not wise to cut our vagus nerves; their job is too important for humans, so we'll have to live with feeling sick when our body is fighting off an infection—for now, at least.[51]

So, while the apostle Paul teaches us to rework our thought patterns,[52] science shows us that doing so will have a direct effect on our health. Unfortunately science also tells us that when we are sick, it will be that little bit harder to ensure our thought patterns are healthy.

Bad thought patterns are also the cause of stress, one of the biggest generators of disease in the western world. Let me explain.

THE TOXIC NATURE OF STRESS

Stress is a state we feel in our minds when the resources we have available aren't enough to meet the demands placed on us at a particular time. Stress can be healthy because it can stimulate us to raise our game but, like any good thing, too much stress is often a problem. We don't just experience stress in our minds, we also experience it in our bodies. When we are stressed, a trigger goes

---

51. The negative aspect of this communication has been observed in cancer patients. Interleukin-1, which is one of the PICs naturally occurring in the body, has been trialed in treating certain cancers. While interleukin-1 has a significant effect on stemming bodily cancer, a side effect that has been consistently noticed is the development of depression in patients who are treated with it, and it is thought this depressive effect occurs through this vagus nerve pathway.
52. See Romans 12:2.

off in our brain, almost like a turbo button in a car, that stimulates our adrenal glands to squirt out a number of hormones into our blood.

Just as a car's engine responds with increased performance when the turbo is pressed, so too, our bodies respond in a similar way. The increased blood levels of epinephrine, norepinephrine, and cortisol cause our hearts to beat faster, releases energy into the blood stream, narrows and focuses our vision, and increases blood flow to our muscles. Physiologists call this the "fight or flight" response, and God has given us this ability to help us out in difficult situations. But if we use it too much, or rely on it to get us through everyday life, then it leads to negative consequences.

A friend of mine owned a two-seater sports car and kindly allowed me to borrow it for a weekend on my first wedding anniversary. Michelle and I loved it. We drove it quite carefully as I wanted to get it back in one piece to my friend, but there was one occasion when, at the bottom of a large hill I put my foot to the floor and felt a click behind the plate. That "click" was the turbo. The engine roared as the car's capacity to take on the steep hill massively increased. I hope my friend agrees that it was a healthy use of the car's turbo. But imagine the state the car would have been in if I floored the gas approaching each traffic light, slamming on the brakes when I got close, and then accelerating off again only to screech to a halt again at the next light. Cars aren't designed to be used this way. And neither are our bodies. This is why psychological stress, without appropriate levels of rest and recovery, is linked to so much ill health.

After a flight or fight response, we should give our bodies time to rest and recover and build up the reserves we have just depleted. But if we go from one stressful moment to the next, not getting adequate rest, then our reserves run low and we don't get time to for the necessary restorative processes. Over time our bodies take strain.

Physiologically, what's happening is that the chronically high levels of cortisol lead to a buildup of the same chemicals (PICs) that produced the sickness response in rats when placed around the rats' brains. PICs have since been implicated in a number of diseases. For instance, their presence seems to irritate the blood vessels around the heart and cause the build-up of cholesterol in the vessels' walls, leading to arterial hardening (atherosclerosis) and heart attacks. Additionally, PICs have also been shown to cause brain degeneration in Alzheimer's and Parkinson's patients and also to be the cause of some cancers (specifically, breast cancer and myeloma).

Increased levels of epinephrine and norepinephrine also have a direct effect on our blood pressure. This is a good thing when we are in danger, because it makes us more alert and ready to fight or run, but if these hormones are constantly present in the background, it seems to keep our blood pressure raised. Prolonged raised blood pressure, as you may know, puts strain on our cardiovascular system and, if untreated, puts us at high risk of strokes later in life.

Another disadvantage of unhelpful stress is that the resulting adrenal hormones disrupt sugar metabolism and cause you to crave junk food. Combined with the high sugar load of Western diets, this risks exhaustion of our pancreas (as the pancreatic cells cannot produce enough insulin to keep up controlling blood sugar levels), and eventually leads to type 2 diabetes, which is growing in epidemic proportions in the Western world. So, cardiovascular disease, hypertension, and type 2 diabetes can all be linked back to stress, a condition that originates in the mind.

THE SPIRITUAL ROOT OF STRESS

As you can see, toxic thoughts and stress produce much ill health. But have you ever thought there might be a spiritual cause underlying this? The answer is that toxic thoughts, stress, and stress-related disease, all have their roots in idolatry. You may think it strange that I refer to idolatry because idolatry is not often a condition Christians are accused of. However, have a look at the last line of John's letter (addressed to Christians): *"Little children, keep yourself from idols"* (1 John 5:21).

I doubt John was worried that New Testament believers would go and carve out wooden statues to worship. Rather, I think he was referring to the situation Ezekiel spoke about when he said the Israelites had *"set up idols in their hearts"* (Ezekiel 14:3 NIV). The Reformer John Calvin expanded on this by saying our heart is an "idol factory," constantly at risk of looking to created things to give us something really only our Creator can give us.

As New York pastor Tim Keller points out, heart idols are not usually things that are inherently bad; they can often be good things.[53] The issue isn't their nature; it's their position. For instance, if our job ceases to be a job but becomes our source of identity or validation, then we have moved into idolatry. We are going to push ourselves to perform beyond our capacity and live in a state of mental stress, hitting our turbo button way too often, and not giving ourselves time for adequate restoration. Likewise, if we determine that our value in life is from how good a parent we are, we are going to push our children to perform and behave unhealthily. As well as straining our relationship with our children, the stress of trying to do this is going to affect our well-being— maybe not right away, but decades of unnecessary mental stress inevitably takes its toll on our health.

Have a look at the story of one of America's most famous billionaires, whose health suffered for years because of the presence of a heart idol.

As a youngster, [John D.] Rockefeller was a strong and husky farm lad. But he drove himself to make money. At thirty-three he was a millionaire; at forty-three he

53. Tim Keller, *Counterfeit Gods* (New York: Dutton, 2009).

controlled the largest business in the world; at fifty-three he was the world's richest person. By then, though, he was but a shell of a man. He developed a condition called alopecia, where the hair falls out. It was said that he looked like a mummy. His income was one million dollars a week but his digestion was so bad that he could eat only milk and crackers. He was despised by many, upon whom he had trampled in his climb to success. He was immersed in anxiety; he could not sleep; he was a wreck. Here was a man whose life seemed over at fifty-three. It was generally agreed that he could scarcely live more than a year or so. Many newspapers already had his obituary on file, ready for his imminent demise.[54]

John D. Rockefeller was a committed member of his local Baptist church and yet it seemed his aggressive worship of money was going unchecked, resulting in a hugely detrimental effect on his health. There are parallels between his situation and the Corinthian church in the first century. There, some of the church members were also caught in serious heart idolatry, and Paul said that their failure to deal with it was also making them sick, even leading to some of their deaths.[55]

While Rockefeller idolized money, something Jesus specifically warned against,[56] the members of the Corinthian church had a different idol: pleasure. But they were pursuing it with the same verve that Rockefeller had done with money.

In Paul's letter to them he said that their gatherings were characterized by selfishness, drunkenness, and infighting.[57] Sexual promiscuity was commonplace and had reached the point where

---

54. Wayne Jackson, "The Curse of Covetousness," *Christian Courier*, https://www. christiancourier.com/articles/1546-curse-of-covetousness-the (accessed 29 May 2015).
55. See 1 Corinthians 11:30.
56. See Matthew 6:24.
57. See 1 Corinthians 11:21; 15:34; 11:18.

one member had sexual relations with his mother-in-law.[58] While their members attended church meetings regularly and claimed to be worshipping God, for many of them it would have been difficult for outsiders to see any difference in their lifestyle from those who worshipped at the pagan temples in the city. This was hedonism cloaked with Christian terminology and ritual.

In living out such flagrant idolatry, Paul said they were drinking judgment on themselves. He said that God was actively allowing their sin to lead to sickness, as a form of discipline, just as a parent may allow a child to live out the consequences of a bad decision, so that they learn their lesson for next time. It is clear that this discipline is different from God's judicial condemnation of sin that all of us were under prior to belief in Christ.[59] In contrast, God's parental discipline is a sign of being a son or daughter.[60]

Paul tried to reason with them, explaining that their failure to examine themselves and confess their sin to God prior to taking communion meant that they weren't actually taking communion.[61] While they were eating bread and drinking wine, and may even have been praying or singing songs to God while they did, they made a mockery of Jesus' costly death by getting drunk and squabbling.

Failure to confess sin, such as heart idolatries, not only harms our relationship with God, it also prevents Him from cleansing us from the effects of that sin, and as Rockefeller and some of the Corinthian church found out, that can result in bodily sickness.[62]

It is not God's heart for His children to live this way and that is why He has sent His Spirit to convict us of sin and its harmful effects.[63] Thankfully for Rockefeller, he responded to this conviction and repented deeply, with quite dramatic results.

---

58. See 1 Corinthians 6:12–20; 5:1
59. See 1 Corinthians 11:29, 32.
60. See Hebrews 12:6.
61. See 1 Corinthians 11:20.
62. See 1 John 1:9
63. See John 16:8.

But very early one morning, as the richest man in the world tossed and turned through another sleepless night, Jesus' words about laying up treasures on earth came to him with a power he'd never felt before…[64] Five hours later John D. Rockefeller climbed out of bed with a new direction in his life. He was now determined, over whatever time might remain, to work as hard at giving his money away as he'd previously worked hard at making it.[65]

Hospitals, universities and Christian missions received millions of dollars from him as he became interested in the poor and the downtrodden. One hundred and twenty years after that life-changing decision, it has been estimated that five hundred million people are alive today because of the discovery of penicillin and the cures for malaria, diphtheria, and tuberculosis that Rockefeller research grants made possible.

As a result of his marvelous change of disposition, something began to occur in the physical life of John D. Rockefeller. He could sleep again. His digestion improved. Rockefeller actually began to enjoy living. And mark this—he did not die at fifty-four, nor even at sixty-four. Rather, he lived to the ripe old age of ninety-eight years![66]

Jesus and the apostle Paul specifically warn us of the danger of idolatry.[67] As John D. Rockefeller repented of this and set his mind instead on seeking *"first the kingdom of God and his righteousness"* (Matthew 6:33), he discovered that his health could be part of the many "things" that got added. Could heart idolatry be contributing to the sickness you are experiencing?

---

64. See Matthew 6:19–21.
65. Steve Murrell, *Equip Training Leaders Manual,* (Manila, Philippines: Every Nation Publishing), 105.
66. Wayne Jackson, "The Curse of Covetousness," *Christian Courier,* https://www.christiancourier.com/articles/1546-curse-of-covetousness-the (accessed 29 May 2015).
67. See Matthew 6:24; 1 Timothy 6:10.

GOD'S COUNTERBALANCE
TO STRESS

While wrong thoughts can lead our body into stress and poor health, the good news is that right thoughts can do the opposite. To mitigate the effects of our bad thought choices, God has built within us a counterbalance that dampens some of the negative health effects. This is why some people can live with potentially unhealthy levels of stress but not suffer the health effects that others suffer. They may not be living as wisely as they could, but they have gained a great advantage by tapping in to this area of God's wisdom and understanding the counterbalance to stress: oxytocin.

Here's what happens: in response to strong empathetic thoughts, a part of the brain called the pituitary gland releases a hormone called oxytocin into the blood. Oxytocin is a wonderful hormone: not only does it dampen down toxic PICs and unhealthy levels of adrenal hormones, but it also releases the neurochemical dopamine, which increases our sense of well-being. This has an additional effect because a sense of positive well-being further dampens down harmful PICs in our body.

Prior to my wife Michelle giving birth to our son JJ, she endured a grueling twenty-three hour labor. Her body was swimming with stress hormones, so one of the first things the midwife did after JJ entered the world was ensure that he was placed next to Michelle to feed. I remember the moment well. Dazed by exhaustion and emotion, Michelle could barely take everything in. But as JJ started to glug down his first meal, Michelle started to cry. With joy lighting up her face she said, "I can't believe it—I am just suddenly so overcome with love for him." Oxytocin was doing its job. Released directly in response to my son's feeding, it was helping an empathetic bond to form and preparing Michelle's body to rest from all the stress it had just gone through.

God has designed all of us to have access to this restorative hormone. When we go through stressful events, He has designed us to connect empathetically with those around us, and our health is rewarded when we do. However, if we are isolated during our stressful times or suffer from regular loneliness, we miss out on the restorative action of oxytocin, and our health may suffer.

For example, parents who stay too long at the office may miss out on that empathetic connection with their children. Spouses who pass like ships in the night likewise miss the chance for the restorative health benefits of taking time out to connect and enjoy each other. Bosses need to be wary when workers become numbers on a spreadsheet, whose sole value is seen in their contribution to the bottom line, because they miss out on the chance to see their employees as God sees them—having intrinsic value outside of their productivity. Those who are sick long-term need be aware of the danger of isolation or of taking those who care for them for granted, because they will start to lose empathetic connection. When we fail to see people as fathers or mothers with families, or as people with hopes and dreams, empathy is lost. Cumulatively, we not only put our relationships at risk, but also our health.

The Bible shows us that God created us for deep connection. That's why He places the lonely in families and why He places us in spiritual families when we become Christians.[68] As well as knowing that this is essential for our spiritual growth, God also knows it has a superb benefit for our health.

While human relationships may let us down, God offers all of us the chance to experience the deepest empathetic relationship in the universe—with Him. The apostle Paul went through the most horrific physical circumstances but he could be joyful because he had learned to connect to God whatever the circumstance.[69] In contrast, Elijah, temporarily, felt isolated from God and was exhausted and miserable, but when God engaged with him he was restored back to health.[70]

---

68. See Psalm 68:6; Acts 2:47.
69. See Philippians 4:12–13.
70. See 1 Kings 19:3–8.

It says in 1 John 4 that *"God is love"* and He lavishes this love on His children. Perhaps some of the sickness we experience stems from failing to connect properly to God, and experiencing that loving, empathetic connection for ourselves. Or perhaps we have failed to connect empathetically with those around us, missing out on the chance to give or receive life-giving words. Our emotional and spiritual choices have huge effects on our health. Proverbs tells us that *"Gracious words are like a honeycomb, sweetness to the soul and health to the body"* (Proverbs 16:24).

Is the sickness you are experiencing related to the mind choices you have made? Have you idolized created things or somehow disconnected from God, and separated yourself from His ability to speak gracious words that bring health to your body?

Toward the end of Paul's long treatise to the Roman church, he encouraged them that a key to living for God in every situation is through renewing one's mind.[71] In other words, changing the way we think not only gives life to our soul but also life to our body.

KEY POINTS:

1. Our thoughts can not only change our experience of sickness but can actually trigger our body to either resist or to succumb to some sicknesses.

2. One of the most dangerous sources of negative effects on our health is excessive stress, which can be rooted in the spiritual condition of heart idolatry.

3. God's powerful counterbalance to stress is oxytocin, a restorative hormone produced when we connect empathetically with those around us. God designed us to be connected with others, and our health is rewarded when we are.

---

71. See Romans 12:2.

CHAPTER 4:

DISCOVERING PURPOSE

"I believe the Scriptures teach that God is aware of every act at every level of the universe. From a star exploding to the rate at which our planet spins to a cell dividing, He knows. I don't believe in the end that God gave me cancer, but He certainly could have stopped it and didn't. So I have to believe like Joseph, John the Baptist, and Paul had to believe when they were in prison—that God is working, and what the enemy means for evil, He will turn to good."

—*Matt Chandler*
Pastor of The Village Church, Flower Mound, TX

At birth Ashleigh appeared to be entirely normal. She was Steve and Pauline's first child, born after just eighteen months of marriage. Like any newborn baby, she had difficulty sleeping, but eventually something much more sinister seemed to appear. Steve and Pauline's worry escalated when, on a couple of occasions, they woke up to find she had stopped breathing. On one occasion, she even turned blue, and they rushed her to the emergency room. There they discovered her windpipe had collapsed, due to a condition called tracheomalacia. Ashleigh spent a month in intensive care and had an experimental procedure performed on her, where her doctors cut vertical lines to create scar tissue to support the windpipe and keep it open.

As she grew, Ashleigh fell further and further behind the normal milestones. Her sleeping was still a big problem, and sometimes she would stay awake for forty-eight hours at a time. Steve and Pauline took her to a number of pediatricians, but nobody could explain what was wrong. They were part of a Bible-believing church, and they felt well-supported by their church community. However, they couldn't help feeling an underlying sentiment from some people that if they had prayed harder as parents, this wouldn't have happened. Up until Ashleigh's first birthday, Steve prayed almost daily for Ashleigh to be healed.

When Ashleigh was two, doctors told Steve that they had discovered demyelination, a condition where the tissue surrounding certain nerves starts to peel away, preventing those nerves from functioning. Her pediatrician predicted she was going to go deaf, then blind, and then die.

This turned out to be incorrect and when Ashleigh was three the same pediatrician suggested she might have a condition called "happy puppets" syndrome. While this diagnosis was being investigated, Steve changed jobs, and inadvertently took with him a floppy disk that had some important files on it. He remembers sitting quietly praying at home one morning at 6 AM, trying to process what was happening with Ashleigh, when the sheriff of the court raided his home, accusing Steve of stealing company secrets.

During this stressful time, Pauline became emotionally involved with another man. She and Steve agreed to go for counseling but after that didn't work out, the church urged Pauline to break off her emotional affair. It was a pressurized time because Steve was in and out of court defending his professional reputation. The financial drain of the court case, the difficulties of looking after a severely disabled child, and the expectations from their church environment became too much for Pauline, and she told Steve she was leaving. A month later she revealed she was pregnant with a child fathered by another man.

While all this was happening the geneticist confirmed that Ashleigh had a severe form of what is now called Angelman's syndrome, a condition caused by the deletion of part of chromosome 15, occurring in every cell in Ashleigh's body.

The diagnosis brought massive relief but also massive pain: relief because the wait was over, but pain because the outcome for Ashleigh was very poor. At that time, Steve told me, only one thousand people in the world had Angelman's syndrome. The condition meant that she would be severely mentally incapacitated and would be wheelchair-bound for the rest of her life.

With his marriage over, and his only child severely disabled, Steve was in crisis. He felt abandoned by God and remembers wistfully saying, "Catch me if you can, God!" In time he left church, started dating, and chose to move in with his girlfriend. Pauline became Ashleigh's fulltime caregiver, and Steve saw her every second weekend. Pauline remarried, and both she and Steve partied hard to try and deal with some of the pain they were feeling.

During this time Ashleigh was regularly hospitalized for various epileptic seizures, a problem that continued until she reached the age of nine. Steve remembers one occasion when the doctors submerged Ashleigh in an ice cold bath to terminate a particularly problematic seizure. Although she couldn't talk, Steve could see that Ashleigh was deeply traumatized by the process, and he remembers holding her in his arms, singing a song over her that calmed her.

After five years of trying to run from God, Steve began to realize that God was patiently pursuing him. He was invited to go on an "Introduction to Christianity" course, and during that time God said to him, "You may have left, but I haven't." Steve was slowly seeing that God was more than up to the challenge of catching people when they challenged Him to do so.

As Steve was being restored by God, he got to know a woman named Lyn at work. Lyn's father had been severely brain damaged after being hit by a truck while walking by the side of the road. He had been unconscious for thirty-six days and now needed full-time caregivers. Lyn's mother also developed Alzheimer's disease, and it was this common understanding of sickness and suffering and their mutual faith in God that led to a five-year blossoming friendship. During this period of friendship they realized they had feelings for each other, so they started dating, which quickly led to marriage.

At the age of ten, Ashleigh was still heavily dependent, requiring round-the-clock care to feed, bathe, and support her, and so Steve arranged for her to be taken into a care facility for severely disabled children. Steve continued his practice of visiting every second weekend, and he could sense a lot of peace in Ashleigh. During this time he twice had a dream of Ashleigh running in a field with Jesus looking on. People with Angelman's syndrome are characteristically very happy, and the only time Ashleigh is ever irritated is when she is in pain or hungry.

In 2014, Ashleigh turned nineteen. She likes to go to the movie theater, and despite not being able to speak, she has an uncanny knack of always knowing where movies are showing in any mall they visit. While her IQ remains equivalent to that of a three-year-old, she recently surprised everyone by learning to walk. When Steve is around Ashleigh, he senses Jesus is very close, and he looks forward to the day when Ashleigh will be with him in heaven and he'll get to hear her talk.

Reflecting back on the last nineteen years, Steve realized that, despite praying for Ashleigh's healing, the real healing has occurred inside of him. As we talked, he became aware that after an eighteen-year gap, he has just started to feel confident to pray for healing again. But this time he's not praying for healing for Ashleigh, but for those God brings to him. Steve loves his daughter dearly and is grateful for way God has worked in his life, realizing that without the changes that happened inside of him through his difficult experiences, he may never have met Lyn.

SPIRITUAL HEALING VERSUS PHYSICAL HEALING

If you are in a position like Ashleigh where your sickness, or the sickness of someone dear to you, came about because of a genetic disease, you may have asked the question, "Why did God allow this sickness to come on me or my loved one?" Knowing that genetic diseases are a result of the fall probably doesn't offer much comfort.[72] While the fall affects everyone, the real question is why have I, or my family, been singled out with this specific, devastating effect? While working in pediatric hospitals, I got to know many children and families who had debilitating diseases, and I know that for many of them, these questions are not abstract concepts but something they wrestle with daily.

As we have said in the early chapters, if we are believers, God permits sickness to occur in our world, for this moment, but, unless we are in massive idolatry, He is not the instigator of our sickness; human sin, folly, or evil is the cause. But if God is all-powerful, why does He permit sicknesses? Nick Vujicic hasn't received an answer as to why he was born with tetra-amelia syndrome. Steve hasn't received an answer as to why God permitted Ashleigh to be born with Angelman's syndrome.

The Bible is clear that God is thoroughly in charge of all that happens in the universe. In Paul's letter to the Colossian church he tells us that Jesus not only created everything, He is also before all things and is currently holding everything in the universe

---

72. See chapter 2 for a detailed discussion on this.

together.[73] Mark tells us that while the disciples witnessed many miracles, they were astounded that the weather was also subject to Him.[74] And Job, realizing the extent of God's involvement in the universe, rhetorically asked, *"Do you know how God controls the clouds and makes his lightning flash?"* (Job 37:15 NIV). Dr. R.C. Sproul sums it up this way:

> If there is one maverick molecule running loose in this universe outside the scope of God's Sovereign authority, power, and control, no Christian has any reason whatsoever to put faith or any trust in any future promise that God has made to His people. For want of a nail the shoe was lost, for want of a shoe the horse was lost, for want of a horse the rider was lost, for want of a rider the battle was lost, for want of a battle the war was lost....One maverick molecule could destroy the best laid plans, not of mice, or of men, but of God, if God is not Sovereign.[75]

Sickness was unleashed by us but, like everything else, it is still under God's sovereignty. D. A. Carson explains the conundrum this way: "To put it bluntly, God stands behind evil in such a way that not even evil takes place outside the bounds of His sovereignty, yet the evil is not morally chargeable to Him: it is always chargeable to secondary agents, to secondary causes."[76]

This is seen in the book of Job, as well; the author is clear that Satan instigated the chaos, but he is also clear that at every point God controlled it and restricted Satan. God could not have done that unless He was fully in control. Through his suffering, Job experienced the promise that Paul penned in his letter to the Romans: that in all things God is working for the good of those

---

73. See Colossians 1:17.
74. See Mark 6:51.
75. R. C. Sproul, from a talk given in Austin, TX (March 9, 1991).
76. D. A. Carson, *How Long, O Lord? Reflections on Suffering and Evil* (Grand Rapids, MI: Baker Academic, 2006), 189.

who love Him.[77] And, as Job discovered, "all" included his sickness. When his friends frustrated him, when his wife gave up on him, God engaged with him and lovingly confronted him.

While the author doesn't fully explain why God allowed these things to happen to Job, we are shown that God used the situation to bring about a deeper and richer relationship with Job and to bring him to a place of greater blessing than before. And it was God's ultimate authority in the situation that placed Him in a position to accomplish Job's complete restoration.

For those of us who suffer, we may, like Job, not get the answers we seek, but we will receive something so much greater than answers—a Person. A Person who is not only in charge, but is pro-health, and perfect in His love for us. A Person who is not only a Person, but also a Father who in the midst of tragedy is working all things for the good of those who love Him; a Father who is working hard to, one day, make His children sickness-free.

Some people have asked, "What is the point of praying to a God who is sovereign over sickness, but who still allows us to receive it?" If you're asking that question, have you considered the alternative? Imagine if sickness wasn't subject to God? What would be the point of praying to a God who couldn't do anything about our situation? Instead of reaping peace through the truth that God is in control and will respond to our request, we would only reap fear and worry. Instead of knowing we have a Father who wanted to and was able to deal with the situation, we'd be like spiritual orphans trying to solve the problem ourselves. And if God had no influence on how it affected us, unlike in Job's case, He wouldn't be able to limit it.

In the 1860s, in industrial Britain, ships were setting sail with dangerously large amounts of cargo. For the ships' owners it was a way to maximize profits because if the ship reached its destination they would be paid more, and if the ship sank, as many of them

---

77. See Romans 8:28.

did, then they could collect insurance money. The people who had the raw end of the deal were the sailors who manned these so-called "coffin ships." Their lives were put in danger by the greed of the ships' owners.

Concerned Christian and member of the UK Parliament Samuel Plimsoll thought something needed to be done. For six years, at times under opposition and ridicule, he campaigned for a line to be painted on ships that would indicate the most a ship could be loaded without jeopardizing safety; because a ship will sink lower in the water the heavier it becomes, and a standard line could indicate safety despite the difference in vessel size. After much political battling he succeeded, and in his honor the standardized safety line was named the Plimsoll Line. It is still a requirement for all ships throughout the world today.

Like Samuel Plimsoll, God too has placed a line on all of us, and, as He did with Job, decreed in the spiritual realm "to here and no more."[78] If we are His followers, His promise to us is that He is, and always will be, faithful, and what He permits will ultimately be worked for our good.

Listen to what John Piper, a person who has experienced the horror of receiving a cancer diagnosis himself, said:

> I have never heard anyone say, "The really deep lessons of
> my life have come through times of ease and comfort." But
> I have heard strong saints say, "Every significant advance
> I have ever made in grasping the depths of God's love and
> growing deep with Him, has come through suffering."[79]

As Nick engaged with God during his difficulties, God dramatically transformed his situation for good. Steve had a longer journey, but God pursued him and reconnected with him. While

---

78. See Job 1:6–12; 2:1–6.
79. John Piper, "Where the Great King Keeps His Wine," DesiringGod.com, November 19, 1990, http://www.desiringgod.org/articles/where-the-great-king-keeps-his-wine (accessed 29 May 2015).

neither Nick nor Steve have received the physical healings they prayed for, what they have both received is emotional and spiritual healings. They have both personally lived through Romans 8:28: "*And we know that in all things God works for the good of those who love him, who have been called according to his purpose*" (NIV).

C. S. Lewis, famed for *The Chronicles of Narnia*, was also a popular speaker. One of his most popular lectures, later turned into a book of its own, was called "The Problem of Pain." Watching his wife die of cancer, he was somebody, like Steve and Nick, who could speak not just intellectually, but also experientially, of the effects of sickness. In his book of the same name, Lewis makes this now-famous statement: "We can ignore even pleasure. But pain insists upon being attended to. God whispers to us in our pleasures, speaks in our conscience, but shouts in our pains: it is His megaphone to rouse a deaf world."[80]

Sometimes we are not even aware that we are spiritually sick, and it takes physical sickness to wake us up. When the blind beggar, Bartimaeus, called out to Jesus, Jesus asked him, "*What do you want me to do for you?*"[81] Bartimaeus might have replied "Jesus, isn't it obvious what I want?—I want to see!" But Jesus is not the sort of person who fails to spot the obvious. Typically His questions are wielded with great penetration and precision. The simplest explanation as to why Jesus was asking Bartimaeus this question is that Jesus had something to offer in addition to physical healing.

If you could swap places with Bart, what would your answer to Jesus be? There is nothing wrong with asking Jesus for healing—rather Jesus is pleased by it—but the wiser question is to say to Jesus, "What healing do I need?"

To paraphrase another quote from C. S. Lewis, the real issue, perhaps, isn't that we pursue healing, it is that we don't pursue

---

80. C. S. Lewis, *The Problem of Pain* (London: The Centenary Press, 1940), 91.
81. Mark 10:51.

healing enough.[82] We may have physical healing on our minds, but Christ has a much deeper and wider healing intent. It seemed this was true for Nick, but it was only when he received emotional and spiritual healing that he was able to make the most of his physical situation. Paul sums up Jesus' heart in this in the final part of his first letter to the Thessalonian church: *"Now may the God of peace himself sanctify you completely, and may your whole spirit and soul and body be kept blameless at the coming of our Lord Jesus Christ"* (1 Thessalonians 5:23).

Jesus doesn't want physical healing only, or spiritual healing only. His desire is for wholeness of our spirit, soul, and body. During His earthly ministry Jesus was very happy for people to approach Him for physical healing, but if you notice, Jesus often addressed something much deeper in the person than the initial request.

When we come to Jesus for healing, He penetrates deep into our heart and sees our ultimate needs. If we ask Him to, Jesus will always come and initiate a healing process, but as our Creator, we need to let Him pick His order of priorities.[83]

To look at one example, if you are suffering from the effects of weighing too many pounds, such as joint aches and difficulty breathing or sleeping, it might be worth looking at whether God wants to bring about change inside of you spiritually, as well physically. Many people view excessive weight gain as purely a physical problem and so try to solve it using purely physical means: trying to increase exercise levels, changing dietary patterns, etc. But with most people, this only brings about mixed results at best,

---

82. In his book *The Weight of Glory* (preached originally as a sermon in the Church of St. Mary the Virgin, Oxford, 8 June 1942; published in *Theology*, November 1931), Lewis wrote, "Our Lord finds our desires not too strong, but too weak. We are half-hearted creatures, fooling about with drink, sex, and ambition, when infinite joy is offered us, like an ignorant child who wants to go on making mud pies in a slum because he cannot imagine what is meant by the offer of a holiday at the sea. We are far too easily pleased."

83. A process that is only completed in believers on the far side of eternity.

particularly over the long term, and it may be more effective to view the issue primarily as a spiritual or emotional issue and only secondarily a physical one.

If you look at animals in the wild, it is not usual for them to regularly take in take more calories than their bodies need, even when they find themselves with an excess of food available. This is because God has placed in animals (and ourselves) mechanisms that prevent excessive intake of calories.[84] For us to eat more calories than we need, we have to suppress these mechanisms, in much the same way that an athlete may suppress the feeling of pain and play on with a damaged knee or shoulder until the game ends.

When I was in my first year of university, I lived in a residence hall that provided three cooked meals a day, included in the monthly rental fee. I remember so enjoying the eggs, bacon, and muffins that were provided each morning that I would sometimes eat past my feeling of fullness, and by so doing, train my body to think that this was ok. I was doing a fair amount of sports at the time, so I justified it to myself by saying that I would use up the extra calories, but I forgot that my body was already telling me how many calories I needed, and I was pushing past this.

Once our body is trained in this way, it is far too easy for us to look to food to fulfill a spiritual function. We may feel a bit down or stressed, and instead of going to God to find some relief, we discover that sugar or fat can provide a temporary solution. We may not be physically hungry, but we are emotionally or spiritually hungry, and we train our body to allow food to fill this gap.

Do you recognize this pattern in yourself at all? Gluttony, or eating beyond hunger,[85] isn't a popular sermon topic but it is probably a big reason why many people gain, and then struggle to

---

84. When we reach a certain threshold of fat or protein our body causes us to feel full. Likewise, once our stomach reaches close to its capacity, stretch receptors in the stomach wall send messages to the brain that we are full. If we eat too much of one food, you may notice that it becomes less and less enjoyable.
85. See Proverbs 28:7; Luke 7:34; and Titus 1:8.

lose, excess weight. God doesn't want us to use food in this way, but the good news is that, if we address the spiritual reasons of why we are, we can begin to change this pattern in our lives, and become healthier. (For more information on why we may not be connecting to God and looking to things like food to fill the void, see chapter 6.)

Spiritual, or inner healing, is a big priority for Jesus, because many of our health issues are rooted at the spiritual level. Having partnered with Jesus in ministering to people for a long time, I am confident to say that if your sickness came about through the actions of others, one of His priorities will be to heal any hurt, bitterness, or shame that you may still feel because of it. Also, if your sickness came as a result of your own unwise actions, then one of Jesus' priorities will be to ensure that you experience His forgiveness. If your sickness is somehow the result of an external evil, then I know that Jesus will want to untangle you from this, and ensure that you are completely free. All of us see the physical manifestations of sickness, but Jesus is the only One who truly sees the whole picture.

There is much wisdom in dealing with inner sicknesses first, because, as we saw in chapter 3, if our mind remains sick then we can open ourselves up to getting physically sick again through a weakened immune system. This can happen even if our sickness was resolved through a dramatic healing. The apostle John alluded to this in his third pastoral letter when he wrote: *"Beloved, I pray that all may go well with you and that you may be in good health, as it goes well with your soul"* (3 John 2).

Here John connects good physical health to good inner health. As we saw in chapter 3, the medical profession is starting to pick up on God's wisdom in this. It's interesting to note that when I was a hospital doctor, the spinal surgeons at one of the hospitals I worked in refused to do back surgery for patients who also had psychological symptoms such as anxiety, depression, passivity, negativity, etc. They found that people with these "yellow flags" did not derive much pain relief from having the surgery. However, if the psychological issues were resolved, the doctors would happily operate, knowing there was a good likelihood of the surgery now deriving benefit. Likewise, a neurosurgeon that I know in Johannesburg advises patients with brain tumors to receive counseling for past hurts, because he has found that this often leads to a big improvement in the person's immune state and, within his practice, at least, increases their chance of cancer survival.

For some, the inner healing God may want to perform during sickness is to bring about spiritual salvation. A pastor I know went to visit one of his church members in the hospital. The man was dying, and after praying for healing, the pastor asked if the man was prepared for death. One of the questions he asked him was, "Are you confident that you will go to heaven when you die?" The man replied that he thought he probably would because during the previous few years he had tried quite hard to live a good life. The man had been in the pastor's church for many years, but it was evident that he had never really grasped the gospel, and so the pastor explained that salvation was not about trying to live a good life. He went on to explain that the man could be confident of his destination without having to rely on his own efforts. This news seemed too good to be, and the sick congregant jumped at the opportunity presented to him. The amazing thing is that it is really true!

Terminal physical illness is rightly seen as a tragedy, but terminal spiritual illness is an infinitely greater tragedy, and if it wasn't for his physical sickness, this man may have missed out on receiving his spiritual healing.

Salvation is not just something God wants to work inside of a sick person. After God healed Nick Vujicic emotionally and spiritually, Nick went on to travel the world, using his situation to tell people about the gospel of Jesus. His physical sickness remained, but it has opened a huge door to bring spiritual healing to many. On one occasion, God permitted Paul to suffer an illness, and although we don't know all the details, we do know that a whole group of people received eternal healing because of it: "*it was because of a bodily ailment that I preached the gospel to you*" (Galatians 4:13).

In his letter to the Galatians, Paul was writing not just to one church, but a group of churches spread across that particular Roman province. That sickness-created opportunity obviously bore fruit because he was now writing to those that responded to his message. At the time Paul may have wondered why his loving God could allow him to experience the specific sickness, but, from the benefit of hindsight, we can see that Paul's sickness resulted in many people coming to know God and receiving surety of their eternal salvation.

If sickness really is a blip on the timeline of God and is something that He will put right—forever—then with so many people around us being threatened with missing out on this beautiful eternity, it is only natural that we would want God to use our situation to reach others. While we may see a world of "physically well" and "physically sick" people and perhaps be despondent that we are in the latter category, God sees the world primarily as people who are "spiritually sick" and people who are "spiritually healed." If we are in God's latter category, then it changes the way we see those who aren't.

SHOULD WE EVEN SEEK PHYSICAL HEALING?

Because of all the ways God can use sickness to bring benefit in us, some have concluded that we mustn't seek physical healing. What really matters, they say, is spiritual healing and spiritual sanctification, and if sickness can carry this out then we should assume that when we get sick, it is God's will for us to remain this way. Taken to its logical conclusion, this error, if believed, would mean that we would never to the doctor for a prescription when we have a bad case of something or go the emergency room to have a broken bone put in a cast. It also has the deeper danger of promoting a dualist philosophy—giving the impression that the spirit is good and the body is bad. In the verse I quoted earlier, John didn't just pray for people's souls, he also prayed for good physical health. Christian theology says that, while currently tainted by sin, both the body and the spirit are good.

Some use the example of Paul's thorn in his flesh to try to back up their argument, but this a misrepresentation of the passage:

> So to keep me from becoming conceited because of the surpassing greatness of the revelations, a thorn was given me in the flesh, a messenger of Satan to harass me, to keep me from becoming conceited. Three times I pleaded with the Lord about this, that it should leave me. But he said to me, "My grace is sufficient for you, for my power is made perfect in weakness." (2 Corinthians 12:7–9)

While Paul certainly seemed to have eye trouble[86] and would have had physical effects from his stonings, whippings, and beatings, the thorn he refers to in his letter is not a physical ailment. The last part of the sentence reveals the nature of the thorn: a "*messenger of Satan.*"

A messenger (someone who brings a message), can't refer to something inanimate such as a sickness. In Scripture, messengers are always living beings of some sort. The most common references to messengers in the Bible are angels (angel literally means "messenger"). A plain reading of the phrase "*a messenger of Satan*" would conclude the messenger to be a fallen angel or demon. An alternative reading interprets Satan's messenger as a human agent because in Joshua 23:13, the Israelites' human enemies are referred to as "*thorns*" in their eyes, and Paul was fond of using Old Testament

---

86. See Galatians 4:15; 6:11.

metaphors in his writings.[87] However it is interpreted, I do not think that the word messenger can credibly refer to a sickness.

In Paul's early letter to the same church he says, *"Do you not know that you are God's temple and that God's Spirit dwells in you? If anyone destroys God's temple, God will destroy him. For God's temple is holy, and you are that temple"* (1 Corinthians 3:16–17). It is Satan, not God, who tries to destroy the bodies of believers (God's temple), with sickness most commonly used as one of his means of destruction. So, while we acknowledge that God can use any sickness we experience for His purposes, this shouldn't distract us from also seeking Him for physical healing.

CAN GOD ONLY HEAL IF SPIRITUAL HEALING HAS OCCURRED?

While I think it is wise to seek inner healing first, we must be careful not to make a rule out of it, because there are plenty of occasions when Jesus heals without mentioning a person's spiritual situation. The psalmist says that *"whatever the LORD pleases, he does, in heaven and on earth, in the seas and all deeps"* (Psalm 135:6), so I am not saying that if you are in a bad spiritual place, God can't or won't heal you. There are many testimonies of God healing people who were very distant from Him and even people from other faith backgrounds. However, in approaching God for physical healing, if you do discover there is something coming between you and Him, why would you not want to do something about it? And in doing so, perhaps it will allow to you experience God's healing grace on your life—not just when Jesus renews all things, but on this side of eternity, too.

Discovering God's purposes in our sickness helps us to keep our focus on God and off our circumstances. In doing so we can access His strength during our period of sickness and we can

---

87. Some have suggested that Alexander the Coppersmith is the messenger of Satan that Paul refers to because of 2 Timothy 4:14–16.

receive His hope for the future. In the next section I'll look at some common blocks that can hinder people from connecting with God, and give some practical steps to remove them. As well as interesting examples and illustrations, each chapter will give an explanation around the theology of the topic and then a chance to put the theology into practice.

An important principle I have discovered is that God often speaks to us about His plans and purposes as we take the first steps. Gathering knowledge is important, but our knowledge needs to lead to action, or it will be of no real benefit. For instance, while Peter and John saw Jesus perform miracles, it was only once they left their fishing nets and journeyed with Him that they learned that He really was the Messiah. The practical elements at the end of the chapters in the next section will help you leave behind some of the hindrances to finding God's purposes in your sickness. The practical suggestions are tried and true, born out of personal experience. As people have applied these principles, I have seen many inner transformations that have sometimes been the key to physical healing.

Don't be like the people who gather all the theory first and plan to go back to the practical steps later. No matter how good their intentions, few people actually do go back and do the practical steps. Rather, I encourage you to interact with these steps as you read them, and not to wait a single moment if you are seeking spiritual and physical healing.

Sometimes these steps will be emotionally tough to do, but I encourage you to press through because of the countless advantages. Here are a few of the advantages for your encouragement:

1. God gives us a blessing when we act in response to His conviction.

All of us want to receive blessings from God, and the apostle James informs us the way to do this is to ensure that we apply what we learn through action: *"being no hearer who forgets but a doer who acts, he will be blessed in his doing"* (James 1:25).

2. We avoid the risk of being deceived.

In contrast to this, James tells us we deceive ourselves if we are convicted, but then don't act on our conviction: *"Be doers of the word, and not hearers only, deceiving yourselves"* (James 1:22).

3. We lay strong foundations in our lives.

In the parable of the wise and foolish builders, both builders hear Jesus' words, but only the wise man builds on a firm foundation to stand against life's storms.[88] Jesus tells us the wise builder does this by putting His words into practice.

4. We can be confident we are learning to be true disciples.

Jesus, when He gave His Great Commission, didn't admonish the disciples to go through the world teaching people to know everything that He commanded them. Rather, Jesus said *"teaching them to **obey** everything that I have commanded you"* (Matthew 28:20 NIV). Knowing without obeying was the trap that the Pharisees fell into. They knew much about what God had said but, by not putting this into practice, they failed to let God's words penetrate their hearts and truly change them. In contrast, we can know that we are following the Great Commission when we obey what Jesus tells us.

KEY POINTS

1. Like everything in the universe, sickness is under God's authority. This enables Him to limit our experience of sickness and be in a position to act when we seek Him for healing.

2. When we do experience sickness, God wants to use our situation to initiate healing—but it is our job to ask Him where He wants to start: in our spirit, soul, or body.

---

88. See Matthew 7:24–27.

3. God's deepest healing is always spiritual, but this shouldn't keep us from seeking God for physical healing also; some may experience physical healing on earth, but if we are spiritually healed all of us will receive complete physical healing in eternity.

SECTION TWO:

REMOVING BLOCKS TO HEALING

"Healing is a matter of time, but it is sometimes also a matter of opportunity."
—*Hippocrates*, Greek philosopher
Author of the Hippocratic Oath

"A healthy outside starts from the inside."
—*Robert Ulrich*
Twentieth-century American actor

"Mental pain is less dramatic than physical pain, but it is more common and also more hard to bear. The frequent attempt to conceal mental pain increases the burden: it is easier to say 'My tooth is aching' than to say 'My heart is broken.'"
—C. S. Lewis, *The Problem of Pain*
Renowned twentieth-century British author

CHAPTER 5:

STOPPING THE BITTER PILL

"The glory of Christianity is to conquer by forgiveness."
—*William Blake*
Nineteenth-century English poet and painter

During the Second World War, Corrie ten Boom, along with her sister Betsie, was sent to the Nazi concentration camp Ravensbrück after they were caught illegally harboring Jews in their home in Amsterdam. Her sister died there, along with the majority of the inmates, but due to an administrative mistake Corrie was released. After the war she went back to Germany as a free woman instead of a prisoner to talk to the German people about forgiveness and reconciliation.

Only two years after the war ended, Corrie was teaching on forgiveness in a room full of solemn-looking Germans. She spoke on God's view of our sin—that once He has forgiven us, He chooses to remember those sins no more. She sensed they were grappling to believe such grace could be really true.

After the talk, a German strode up to her. To her horror, Corrie recognized him as one of the guards at Ravensbrück. As he walked toward her, Corrie had a flashback. She could picture him wearing his Nazi guard's uniform, with its black symbol, and then her feeling of shame as she filed past him naked in a line of prisoners. She remembered her sister, Betsie, with frail bones sticking out of an emaciated body, walking ahead of her.

The ex-guard thanked her for her talk and for explaining the miracle of forgiveness. He obviously didn't remember Corrie, but she certainly remembered him—one of the harshest guards at the camp. He told her that he had since become a Christian and how grateful he was that all his sins from back then had been forgiven, but he stated that it would mean a lot to him if Corrie could speak those words of forgiveness over him. Her response was, at first, utter disgust.

> It could have been many seconds that he stood there— hand held out—but to me it seemed hours as I wrestled with the most difficult thing I had ever had to do.
>
> For I had to do it—I knew that. The message that God forgives has a prior condition: that we forgive those who have injured us. *"If you do not forgive others their trespasses,"* Jesus says, *"neither will your Father [in heaven] forgive your trespasses"* (Matthew 6:15). And still I stood there with the coldness clutching my heart...
>
> "Jesus, help me!" I prayed silently. "I can lift my hand. I can do that much. You supply the feeling." And so woodenly, mechanically, I thrust out my hand into the one stretched out to me. And as I did, an incredible thing took place. The current started in my shoulder, raced down my arm, sprang into our joined hands. And then this healing warmth seemed to flood my whole being, bringing tears to my eyes.
>
> "I forgive you, brother!" I cried. "With all my heart!"
>
> For a long moment we grasped each other's hands, the former guard and the former prisoner. I had never known

God's love so intensely, as I did then. But even then, I realized it was not my love. I had tried, and did not have the power. It was the power of the Holy Spirit.[89]

As Corrie's story shows us, forgiveness isn't easy. Even though most of us will never have to forgive such offenses as a Nazi guard's cruelty in a concentration camp, we still sense something in us that resists the process of forgiveness, no matter how small the offense. But, as we saw in Corrie's story, if we overcome the resistance, there is much to gain.

I have sat with many people and assisted them in forgiveness. Consistently, once they manage to forgive at a deep level, they always remark that they feel so much lighter. It is as though a burden is lifted or as if a tie holding them to the person or situation is broken, and they are able to move on with their lives. This is the problem with unforgiveness and bitterness—they both hold us back, even sometimes holding us back from receiving healing.

One person I prayed for in my church had osteoarthritis in both knees and his lower back. As I prayed for his back, I felt the area get warm, and he reported an instantaneous pain relief that remains to this day. However, when I went to pray for his knees, there seemed to be something blocking the healing power that I felt on my hands. I quickly prayed to God for guidance, and I got the sense that unforgiveness was at play.

I asked the person I was praying for to pause for a moment and tell me if there was anyone he might need to forgive. He initially couldn't think of anyone, but then, as we asked the Holy Spirit to bring people to mind, he realized that he might still need to forgive his two sisters. I guided him through forgiving his siblings, and I then recommenced praying for healing. This time he obtained instant relief. The next week I found him kneeling during the service. I asked him afterwards how his knees were. He told me he was amazed at the depth of the healing, because he hadn't been able to kneel in years.

89. Corrie Ten Boom, "I'm still learning to forgive," *Guideposts*, 1972.

The link between unforgiveness and physical healing runs quite deep. The apostle James simply states: *"Confess your sins to one another and pray for one another, that you may be healed"* (James 5:16). When Jesus healed the paralytic man, He forgave his sins and then commanded him to get up and walk.[90] In receiving forgiveness from the sins, the man received his physical healing without even being prayed for. Derek Prince tells of a similar experience that a Christian psychiatrist had:

> While visiting a hospital, he met a woman who was in a hopeless condition. Her kidneys had ceased to function, her skin was discolored, and she was in a coma, simply waiting to die. One day, he was prompted by the Holy Spirit to say, "In the name of the Lord Jesus Christ, I remit your sins," later wondering if he had done something foolish. About a week later, he was amazed to see the woman walking down the street—completely healed. Unforgiven sin had caused her physical condition. When her sins were forgiven through this man's intercession, her spirit was clear with God and the way was open for her to be healed.[91]

Unforgiveness causes us much trouble and can prevent us from accessing God's grace.[92] As we have seen, this can be from failing to receive forgiveness from God or from failing to forgive others.

UNDERSTANDING FORGIVENESS[93]

If forgiving is something that is so good for us to do but so bad for us when we don't, why do we not do it more often? In Matthew

90. See Luke 5:17–26.
91. Derek Prince, "April 5—Healing Through Forgiveness," Derek Prince Ministries, http://www.derekprince.org/Articles/1000120806/DPM_US/Resources/Daily_Devotional/Daily_postings/April_05_Healing.aspx (accessed 29 May 2015).
92. See Hebrews 12:15.
93. I would like to acknowledge Neil Anderson and Steve Goss for a number of concepts in this chapter that are drawn from their talk, "Forgiveness from the Heart" in the Freedom in Christ course. www.ficm.org.uk

18:21–22, we pick up on Peter wrestling through the idea of forgiveness: *"Then Peter came up and said to him, 'Lord, how often will my brother sin against me, and I forgive him? As many as seven times?' Jesus said to him, 'I do not say to you seven times, but seventy-seven times.'"*

Some say that Jesus picked number seventy-seven in order to contrast with Lamech's declaration in Genesis 4:24: *"if Cain's revenge is sevenfold Lamech's is seventy-sevenfold."* World history is full of examples of people following Lamech's disproportionate vengeance. World War I is a tragic example of this. It was triggered by an assassination of the heir to the Austro-Hungarian Empire by a terrorist group. The resultant ultimatum given by the Austro-Hungarian Empire to the kingdom of Serbia resulted in a war where nine million combatants and seven million civilians lost their lives.

What would our world be like if our paradigm was changed to where we followed Jesus' example when others wrong us? Instead of living in a world with escalating patterns of vengeance, what if we lived in a world of escalating patterns of forgiveness? Jesus follows on from Peter with this parable:

> *Therefore the kingdom of heaven may be compared to a king who wished to settle accounts with his servants. When he began to settle, one was brought to him who owed him ten thousand talents. And since he could not pay, his master ordered him to be sold, with his wife and children and all that he had, and payment to be made. So the servant fell on his knees, imploring him, "Have patience with me, and I will pay you everything." And out of pity for him, the master of that servant released him and forgave him the debt.*

> *But when that same servant went out, he found one of his fellow servants who owed him a hundred denarii, and seizing him, he began to choke him, saying, "Pay what you owe."*

So his fellow servant fell down and pleaded with him, "Have patience with me, and I will pay you." He refused and went and put him in prison until he should pay the debt. When his fellow servants saw what had taken place, they were greatly distressed, and they went and reported to their master all that had taken place.

Then his master summoned him and said to him, "You wicked servant! I forgave you all that debt because you pleaded with me. And should not you have had mercy on your fellow servant, as I had mercy on you?" And in anger his master delivered him to the jailers, until he should pay all his debt. So also my heavenly Father will do to every one of you, if you do not forgive your brother from your heart. (Matthew 18:23–35)

We see in this parable a number of things:

There is a man with an impossible debt. Jesus uses the figure of ten thousand talents to represent something way beyond anybody's reach. Putting things in perspective, King Herod the Great's annual revenue from his entire kingdom was about nine hundred talents, less than 10 percent of this figure.[94]

The man asks to be given time to pay it off. Knowing the value of a talent, the initial hearers would know this would be an absolute impossibility for anyone. The king, in a magnificent gesture of mercy, forgives him the entire debt—and it is understood by the hearers that the king will have to fund the debt from his own resources.

But the man doesn't get what's happened. He fails to let this event change him, and rather than follow in his king's footsteps, he instead does the exact opposite. Later he finds himself in the same position as the king, and his colleague who owes him makes exactly the same plea that he previously made: "Give me more time and I'll pay it off." But his colleague's debt is miniscule in comparison with his own. Matthew

---

94. S. J. Kistemaker, *The Parables* (Grand Rapids, MI: Baker Books, 2002, 2nd ed.), 66.

tells us that one denarius was a day's wage for a laborer,[95] so a servant of the king should have been easily able to pay off this debt.

Instead of being merciful, the first servant demands instant justice and puts his colleague in debtor's prison. In vast contrast to the attitude of the king, he doesn't even grant the plea for more time to pay. When the king finds out, he reverses his decision and puts the servant in prison instead, freeing the other servant.

Do you spot who you and I are in the parable?

We do this all the time. People hurt us or upset us, and, forgetting how God let us off an impossible debt, we put those who hurt us in prison—not an actual prison, but an emotional prison; we cut them off from our families and friends, and if we do speak with them, it is often devoid of any emotional warmth.

We may feel in control of the situation by putting those who hurt us in an emotional prison, but the parable points out that by so doing, we are actually losing control. We are placing ourselves in prison—the person who feels the real negative effects of our unforgiveness is ourselves! The Irish-American actor Malachy McCourt famously sums it up this way: "Resentment is like taking poison and waiting for the other person to die." The eighteenth-century English poet Samuel Johnson said: "A wise man will make haste to forgive, because he knows the true value of time, and will not suffer it to pass away in unnecessary pain."

Nobody wants to suffer in unnecessary pain, so at the end of the parable Jesus tells us the solution to avoid this: we need to follow the king's example and forgive the debt completely, forgiving the other person "*from your heart*" (Matthew 18:35).

HEART-LEVEL FORGIVENESS

When there is forgiveness at the level of the heart, it leads to real heart change—as Corrie ten Boom discovered. Sometimes

95. See Matthew 20:2.

we can think we have forgiven, but if our feelings haven't changed, it is unlikely that we have forgiven deeply enough. I have helped many people to do this deep-level forgiveness and it is not always as straightforward as you may think. For instance, I was once asked to meet with someone who was struggling with not wanting to see his father. His father had left the family while he was very young, and he still felt aggrieved by this. The person informed me he had forgiven his father, but when I chatted with him it became apparent that he still had a lot of anger toward him.

I asked him to close his eyes and picture his father and then describe what emotions came to mind. He listed off anger, bitterness, abandonment, coldness, etc., and I knew a deeper level of forgiveness needed to occur. The author Lewis B. Smedes said, "You will know that forgiveness has begun when you recall those who hurt you and feel the power to wish them well." Robert Muller, former Assistant Secretary General of the UN said: "To forgive is the highest, most beautiful form of love. In return, you will receive untold peace and happiness."

Since this person was experiencing bitterness and coldness, rather than peace and happiness, I managed to persuade him that things could be different. I taught him how to forgive from the heart, with the result that all his negative feelings changed. His feelings were replaced with the same feelings God would have toward the man's father. He discovered what many before him have discovered: the issue wasn't in his feelings, but in his heart.

How does this work? Well, just as our nerves tell us the state of our body, our feelings tell us the state of our heart. So, just as pain in our finger tells our brain that there is something wrong in our finger (it's touching a hot pan, the skin has been cut, etc.) so negative feelings inform us there is something amiss in our heart.

You may be surprised to learn that in the same way that pain is neither morally good nor bad, our feelings are not inherently good or inherently sinful, either. Rather, it is the motivations of the heart that add the moral component to our feelings. For instance, jealousy is often thought of as negative emotion but it can also be positive: Paul said he felt a divine jealousy for the Corinthian church, and God frequently told of His jealousy for Israel.[96] Whether the feeling of jealousy is good or bad depends on the person's motive. When a jealous emotion is present, it should trigger us to realize there is something going on in our heart. Knowing this, we can then explore our heart to see if it is good or bad jealousy.

Graham's Story

Graham hung around after our young adults meeting and mentioned he had gout and arthritis that had been confirmed by a recent scan. I examined his right thumb and as I moved the joint we both heard the loud crackles as the gouty crystals resisted normal movement of the bending joint. In prayer I commanded the gout to go, but as I was doing so, I felt God say that he needed to forgive someone first. I asked him if this was true, and he said he knew he needed to forgive his mom. I turned on my laptop and took him to this chapter and talked him through the process. Following the method at the end of the chapter, he forgave his mom from his heart, and his feelings quickly followed. When he checked the emotion he had toward her, he was surprised to see that he no longer had the feeling of bitterness toward her but all that remained was love. We didn't even need to return and pray for his thumb because simply by carrying out true heart forgiveness, the joint became fully mobile and pain free. I examined the joint again and there was a full range of movement and the crackling sound had completely disappeared. It remains so to this day.

After we saw the pain in Graham's thumb joint resolve I asked him if he had any more pain currently. He said

96. See 2 Corinthians 11:2; Deuteronomy 4:24; Joshua 24:19; and Joel 2:18.

he was experiencing pain in both his knees. I started to pray for this pain also but again I sensed he needed to forgive somebody. After Graham asked the Holy Spirit, a few more people came to mind. I took him through the steps again, and this time when I prayed for his knees the pain instantly went away. Graham also remarked that his jaw was clicking whenever he moved it. I examined it and found the muscles around his jaw were incredibly tight. We spent a moment asking the Holy Spirit if there was a spiritual cause to this, and I felt this was something to do with control. He shared that, growing up, his mother had been very controlling toward him. He forgave his mother for this, and his jaw loosened a little. I then led him to forgive others who had tried to control him in his life, and as he did so, I sensed he had a fear of being controlled by people. As he repented of this, his jaw returned to normal. He told me later that he spent the next few days waggling his jaw, amazed at how mobile it now was. The clicking also went away. Remarkably, all his physical symptoms were healed as he forgave from the heart.

Take joy as another example. Joy is generally considered a positive emotion, but have you ever seen occasions when somebody is joyful at somebody else's demise?[97] On this occasion the joy seems to be negative, and it is because an underlying negative motive has been detected in the person's heart.

There is a lot of confusion about this topic because the English language uses some words to represent both the feeling and the underlying motive. For instance, lust is often considered a feeling, but it is actually a combination of a feeling (sexual arousal) combined with a motive (selfish intent). The feeling is morally neutral, but the motive is not.

---

97. Psychologists refer to this type of joy by the German word *Shadenfreude*, an unhealthy happiness at seeing others fail.

If we can separate feelings from motives we can see that pure feelings act as the thermometer of our heart. They tell us our heart's temperature. When we forgive at this level, we deal with the underlying issue and our feelings follow suit. We see this from Jesus' parable. According to the parable, unforgiveness puts us in prison. When we forgive, we are released from that prison and will inevitably feel differently. If you are feeling a lot of negativity toward people, and you realize that it is affecting you, you may still be in prison. The solution is to learn to forgive from your heart.

So, how do we carry out heart-level forgiveness?

To do so we first have to understand what forgiveness is *not*. There are six common misconceptions I have found about forgiveness that are barriers to true heart-level forgiveness.

1. Forgiveness is not reconciliation.

Reconciliation is returning back to a former, healthier state of relationship. A lot of people are held back from forgiving because they confuse forgiveness with reconciliation. After forgiveness, reconciliation may happen or it may not. Steve Murrell, the co-founder of the group of churches I am part of, said this: "Forgive always, but only restore relationships to the level of repentance."

Forgiveness is an essential first step to reconciliation, but there are other things that need to happen before reconciliation can occur—and it may not always be appropriate to reconcile. For instance, somebody who was injured by an unknown attacker would need to forgive the person for the injury that was caused, but there is no requirement for reconciliation, because there was no relationship in the first place.

A person should forgive an abusive spouse, but if there is no repentance from the spouse, reconciliation shouldn't happen until there is, and trust is re-earned. Trust is a precious commodity, and after it has been broken it needs to be rebuilt slowly. Jesus wants us to distinguish between being innocent and being naïve.[98] We are innocent when we forgive at the earliest opportunity and prevent bitterness from springing up. Because our feelings change we often feel like reconciling; however, we would act naively if we went back in an abusive situation without confirmed and demonstrable heart change by the previous abuser.

2. Forgiveness is not about being the better person.

The motivation to forgive comes from the realization that our own debt also was truly unpayable and that the only option for us was mercy or eternal imprisonment. It is my hope that at some point, like me, you realized there was no way you could have ever paid off the debt you owed to God and that, like the man in the parable, you needed to fall on Jesus' mercy. In response to this, Jesus declares our debt paid. The reality is that if you don't really feel or think that you need much forgiveness from Jesus, then you will struggle to forgive others.

I once counseled a man named James who told me that he had led a pretty decent life; he could see why his friends needed God's mercy but he couldn't really see why he needed it. Knowing how much the Spirit loves to bring truth I suggested that we pray and ask God to reveal if this was true. As he closed his eyes he saw a representation of his good deeds stacked up. His pile was bigger than his friends' but as he zoomed out he saw that his deeds were pathetically short of God's requirement. The more he zoomed out he saw that the difference that he could see between him and his friends seemed less and less until, in comparison with Jesus' perfection, they all looked exactly the same, all dwarfed by Jesus' deeds that actually reached the incredibly high requirement set by God.

After this, James saw another picture in his mind, a picture of him hammering the nails into Jesus' hands on the cross. It dawned on him how proud he had been, and how even that pride was

---

98. See Matthew 10:16.

something that Jesus had to die for. I led him through a prayer of repentance, which enabled him to connect to God better.

Like James, we need to understand the mercy God has made available to us. When we do, we'll find it easier to show others mercy. As the man in the parable found out, it just doesn't make sense to escape justice ourselves and then demand it to rain upon others.

3. Forgiveness is not denying wrongdoing nor is it pretending the situation didn't happen.

When you forgive, you cancel the debt that was owed, but that doesn't mean there wasn't a debt in the first place. I find that people often feel obligated to follow God's example in "remembering sins no more" before true forgiveness happens, and this is a big hindrance to heart-level forgiveness.

In contrast to this, I have found that effective forgiveness only really happens when we see the full horror of the debt that is owed to us. By forgiving, we absorb the debt, and we give up the right to demand justice or treat people badly, but we never deny that what they did was wrong or evil. Amazingly, what happens when we forgive well is that the pain of the situation goes away and, as time goes by, even the memories of the situation seem to fade. Remembering sins no more is not something we have to work at—it seems to occur naturally (when we have forgiven at the heart level).

My wife Michelle had something happen to her as a child that required a lot of prayer and counseling to work through. Since that time she has forgiven the relative who caused it, and they have reconciled well. To see them hanging out today you wouldn't imagine that anything negative had occurred in the past. She forgave well, from the heart; her feelings changed, and the pain went away.

4. Forgiveness is not a feeling.

Forgiveness is a choice. It's an act of obedience to Jesus; an act of worship. Nobody feels like forgiving—ever. Forgiving is emotionally hard to do; it is not easy, particularly if you are not used to keeping short accounts.[99] The longer the hurt has been there, generally, the harder it will be to forgive, but we still need to.

It has been said that time heals all wounds, but that has not been my experience. Having seen enough wounds in the emergency department, I know that wounds heal when all the dirt is cleaned out of them and any infection is treated. It is the same emotionally. Wounds heal when they are appropriately dealt with. Time dulls the pain a little, but if the wound is still there, when somebody touches the spot, it will still hurt!

Have you ever been on the receiving end of somebody's intense anger, and you couldn't understand why? While you may have done something to hurt that person, you were probably confused by how the person's response seemed disproportionately intense compared to the small offense you committed. If that was the case, you probably touched an emotional wound that hadn't properly healed, and you are reaping the pain that somebody sowed before you.

Forgiveness is a choice, and if we forgive fully, from the heart, the pain goes away, because Jesus heals the wound. The great news is that the more people you forgive, and the more frequently you forgive, the easier it gets, and as you get healed of your wounds you won't blow up so much or react so impulsively.

5. Forgiveness is not letting people off.

In the parable it cost the king to forgive. And it cost Jesus to forgive us; He absorbed our debt. Likewise, it costs us to forgive. When a child is born with cerebral palsy due to a mistake by the obstetrician or midwifery team, the family has to bear the cost every day of raising a severely disabled child; things that should take minutes sometimes take hours.[100] The child has to bear the

---

99. See Ephesians 4:26–27.
100. Cerebral palsy can develop in a variety of ways during pregnancy, birth, and early childhood. Some cases have been attributed to mistakes made by health professionals during birth and is part of the reason why malpractice insurance is commonly very high for those who are involved in labor and delivery.

cost of not being able to do all that he or she may have done because the disability has severely narrowed his or her options.

Somebody has to pay the cost, but with forgiveness you say, "They owe me, but I'll pay." And in so doing, you get the opportunity to act like God; to not do the human thing, but, instead, do the divine thing. You get the chance to offer mercy instead of justice, and as you do so you are acting as a true child of our Father in heaven: *"But love your enemies, and do good, and lend, expecting nothing in return, and your reward will be great, and you will be sons of the Most High, for he is kind to the ungrateful and the evil. Be merciful, even as your Father is merciful"* (Luke 6:35–36).

Would you like God to refer to you as a "son [or daughter] of the Most High"? When we forgive, we are demonstrating our heavenly family likeness. While it seems as though the other person gets the better end of the deal when we forgive, we don't forget about justice; we just entrust it to somebody else. Romans chapter 12 says it's God's responsibility to ensure those who hurt us get their due, and ultimately God will sort out the justice of it. On judgment day either they, like us, will be forgiven by Jesus, or they will be held accountable for everything by Jesus. Jesus will be the just Judge. Our job is to forgive. And as we forgive, we unlock the door to our prison and all the benefits freedom contains.

6. Forgiveness is not listening to someone saying sorry.

While listening to somebody apologizing or repenting is a good thing, forgiveness is more than that. We have to go the next step and declare the person forgiven. Forgiveness is always active. It is something we do, a choice we make. This leads us to the next section.

A PRACTICAL WAY TO FORGIVE FROM THE HEART

As I said at the end of the previous chapter, please don't be tempted to skip the practical part. Even if you don't feel you need to forgive anyone, go through the first step and God may surprise you.

This is the method that I have found to consistently work. While I'll demonstrate with a trivial example to show how God cares about forgiving even the small things, I have used this method successfully with people who have gone through the most horrific of circumstances. The freedom, however, isn't in the method but in the heart-level forgiveness. If you have found a different way to do it, great! If you haven't, then why not try this approach? Some people may find it helpful to have a friend present as you got through this process.

STEP A: SETTING THE SCENE

+ Choose a place where you won't be disturbed.

+ Choose a moment when you will not be interrupted.

+ Turn off your cell phone.

+ Grab a pen, paper, and a willing heart to respond to God.

STEP B: DISCOVER WHO YOU NEED TO FORGIVE

+ Take a blank piece of paper.

+ Ask God to bring to mind those whom you need to forgive.

+ It can be helpful to divide the paper into "childhood," "teen-age years," "twenties," etc. if you haven't completed this step before.

+ Write down the names of people (or groups of people) that come to mind, even if you don't feel as though you need to forgive them or feel as though you have already forgiven them. For some people it will be obvious whom you need to forgive, but for others you may be surprised whom the Holy Spirit brings to mind. When I did this exercise, one of the people the Holy Spirit brought to mind was a classmate from my middle school whom I rarely thought about. But when I did reflect on it, I realized I couldn't help having a negative feeling whenever something reminded me of him, and I realized that the Holy Spirit probably knew what was going on in my heart far better than I did.

STEP C: IDENTIFY THE SPECIFIC SITUATIONS

+ Choose one of the easiest people first and write that person's name down on the top of a piece of paper.

+ Ask God to bring to mind the specific instances that you need to forgive.

+ Write down the situations that come to mind and be as specific as possible, e.g. "the time when they said _____ or did _____."

+ When you have your list, ask God to give you the strength to forgive.

Note: It is in forgiving the specifics that we forgive well. Saying, "I forgive _____ for everything they did to me" has, in practice, proven far less penetrating than taking the time to forgive specific incidents where the people hurt you. With my example of the middle school classmate, I followed the process and asked the Holy Spirit about the specifics, and I was reminded of an incident when we had identical pens. He broke his and switched his with mine. I didn't do anything about it at the time because he was the class bully, but the injustice of it quietly gnawed away at me for a time.

STEP D: THE FORGIVENESS PRAYER

+ Take the first instance on your list.

+ Try to remember the pain of the situation. See the sin committed against you for what is was—don't minimize it or underplay what happened.

+ When you feel you are ready, declare out loud: "I choose to forgive _____ for (state the specific instance)." Make sure you say words like, "I choose to forgive." I have had people pray prayers like, "God please help me to forgive..." While that is fine, it isn't actually forgiving. Forgiveness is a choice we make. So I always encourage them by saying, "Great prayer, now proceed to the next step and say, 'I choose to forgive...'"

+ Once you have done this, cross off the instance on the paper.

+ Repeat with the next instance until all the instances have been crossed off.

+ Don't rush; go at a pace that suits you. If it brings up a lot of emotions, pause and ask God for strength, then carry on.

+ When you have crossed off everything on your list, ask the Holy Spirit if there are any more instances.

+ If there are, write them down and repeat the process for these ones until you feel there is nothing left that God wants you to forgive.

STEP E: DOUBLE-CHECKING HEART-LEVEL FORGIVENESS

+ When you think you have forgiven every instance, close your eyes and picture the person. What emotions or thoughts come to mind when you think of the person?

+ Write down the feelings that come to mind. (Be honest with yourself. Sometimes we try to manufacture the right feelings, but it is better to get the honest feelings.)

+ If you have forgiven fully, you should start to feel the same way about the person that God does: this could be sadness about the person's sin and sadness about what has happened, but also some love for them, wanting them to connect better with God.

+ If you still have some negative feelings, go back to Step C and see what other things you need to forgive. (You may need to be more specific if you have been too general.)

+ Once your feelings come into line with how you'd expect God to feel about them, double-check your heart by choosing to pray for the person.

+ Pray for the person to connect with God and, if he or she is not a believer, to become a believer. If there is still reticence in your prayer it is likely that you still have things to forgive and you should go back to Step C.

+ Once you have completed this, repeat the process for everyone on your list. It is ok if you don't finish this all in one go, but make sure you plan a time to go back and finish. Remember, the effects of forgiveness only kick in when you actually forgive!

+ What you have just done is show mercy instead of demanding justice. The reason that I suggest praying for the people you forgave is that as followers of Jesus we have the privilege of stepping beyond mercy—rather than just not giving people what they deserve, we get to give people things they don't deserve. This is grace. A first step in giving people grace is to pray for them. Jesus told us to pray for our enemies,[101] and the person you have just forgiven, has, in effect been your enemy. You will know you have really forgiven from your heart when you are able to pray for that person's good.

SOME FREQUENTLY ASKED QUESTIONS:

+ What if my name is on the list? Do I forgive myself?

If you are one of the people on the list (i.e. you feel as though you need to forgive yourself), I'd suggest phrasing it as repentance before God, rather than forgiveness. For example, if you feel you need to forgive yourself for messing up then say: "God, I am sorry for messing up and the consequences it caused," and then list them.

+ What if my feelings don't change?

If your feelings don't change, this usually means there is more forgiveness to do and possibly you need to be more specific. I find that forgiveness is like peeling an onion. Every layer you peel off is helpful in getting to the core. Some people can get to the core straight away, but others have some layers to peel off first.

---

101. See Matthew 5:44.

+ How should I end the process?

At the end of the process I'd recommend saying sorry to God for holding onto unforgiveness, and not forgiving sooner.

+ What if I just don't feel at all?

There seems to be a situation when people are hurting so much that they decide that, rather than feel the hurt, it is better not to feel at all. I refer to this as carrying out an emotional shutdown, because, while it does stop the hurt (to some extent), it also stops all the positive feelings one can feel. It is as though you are emotionally numb or hardened.

As a child I thought it would be great if I could somehow stop feeling pain. If I fell out of a tree, it wouldn't hurt anymore! The idea held appeal until I came across the disease leprosy, which does exactly that. The bacteria attack the nerves in the hands and feet, and the victims stop feeling pain. The problem is that without pain receptors, those with leprosy have no way of knowing when they touch something hot by accident. Most people with untreated leprosy lose many of their fingers and toes because, without feeling pain, they accidently burn themselves over and over again, each time destroying a bit more of their hands and feet.

Shutting down your emotions comes with a cost, too, but usually at the expense of other people. If this has happened to you, just ask Jesus to reverse what has happened. Say sorry for shutting down your emotions and all the effects that has had on others. Even if you don't seem to feel much, you can still go through the forgiveness steps—but rather than imagining the person and sensing if your feelings change, rather, pray for the person, to see if you have forgiven from the heart. If you are able to genuinely pray for their good, then you have probably forgiven from the heart. If forgiveness has been a real struggle for a long time you may need to read the chapter on fear, sexual sin, and the occult, and then come back to this chapter.

KEY POINTS

1. Failing to receive forgiveness from God or failing to forgive others can directly affect our health and also our ability to access God's healing.

2. We can forgive at different levels, but to experience the health benefits forgiveness brings us, we need to forgive at the level of our heart.

3. A sign that we have carried out heart-level forgiveness is when our feelings toward a person change for the good.

CHAPTER 6:

UNTANGLING LIES

"And so we came forth, and once again beheld the stars."
—*Dante Alighieri, The Divine Comedy*

In December 1944, Lieutenant Hiroo Onoda of the Imperial Japanese Army was sent to Lubang Island in the Philippines. As an intelligence officer he was told to gather information and conduct guerrilla warfare against the locals. He was given the strictest instructions that under no circumstances was he to surrender or take his own life. On arriving on the island he joined up with the Japanese soldiers that were already there, but after the Allied invasion, the group dwindled to only four soldiers, so he ordered them to head to the hills.

Nine months later the emperor of Japan surrendered to the Allied forces, and the Second World War was over. The Japanese army tried to inform Onoda and his team that the war had finished, but their efforts failed. The first set of leaflet drops arrived in October, two months after the Japanese surrender, ordering all Japanese soldiers to give themselves up, but Onoda and his small band of soldiers deemed them to be fake, due to the large number of obvious errors they contained.

The four of them carried on their "war" for four more years until one of the group became separated from the others. After six months of surviving in the hills alone, the separated soldier gave himself up. The loss of one of their members hardened their resolve, and they decided to carry on fighting.

In 1952, seven years after the war had finished, letters and pictures from their families were airdropped to the three remaining soldiers, but again they considered this to be a trick of the enemy. They survived by foraging for bananas and coconuts and by stealing cattle from the local farmers— this was war after all, they reasoned. In 1954, another of their number died in a skirmish with some of the locals, no doubt in response to their thievery. Things went quiet thereafter, and so five years later, back in Japan, Onoda's name was added to the war dead.

Onoda and his fellow soldier carried on, oblivious that the world around them was now a much different place. When news about the 1964 Olympics filtered through to them they considered it odd that Japan was competing alongside the United States, but they reasoned that if the war really were over, they would have received new orders by now. Eight years later, in 1972, while burning rice as part of their continued guerrilla activity, Onoda's final colleague was killed by police. The police, realizing Onoda must be still be alive, arranged for a search party to be sent out to find him, but again this attempt was unsuccessful. Now all alone, Onoda thought the only option open to him was to carry on.

Finally, in 1974, Norio Suzuki, a former Japanese student who had aspirations of being an explorer, found Onoda in the hills of Lubang. Onoda held a rifle to him, but very calmly Suzuki said, "Onoda-san, the emperor and the people of Japan are worried about you." He told him the war was over, but Onoda replied that he would need this to be confirmed by his commanding officer, as his previous orders were under no circumstance to surrender, and he needed new orders before he could stop following the old ones.

The student returned to Japan and, amazingly, found Onoda's war-time commanding officer, retired Major Yoshimi Taniguchi, now working as a bookseller. Suzuki brought the retired major to the island.

So, on the ninth of March, 1974—almost twenty-nine years after the end of the war—at the order of Major Taniguchi, Onoda surrendered. He presented himself in his thirty-year-old army uniform (which had more patches than original material) and turned in his rifle, five hundred rounds of ammunition, his Samurai sword, and the knife his mother had given him (to commit suicide with should he be captured).

At last Onoda knew the truth that the Second World War was over, and he could return home.[102]

⌒

Living with false beliefs, no matter how sincerely held, creates relational blocks that can be costly. For Onoda, his belief that the Second World War was still carrying on meant that he missed out on seeing his family for thirty years! Worse still, two of his colleagues died without ever seeing their friends and families again.

Likewise, if we don't live in the truth, it can create a relational block, and it is extremely dangerous to our health when this relational block is between God and us. Like Onoda, sometimes a false belief can feel so true that it is difficult to believe anything else. Onoda was still wearing his army uniform, and he was still fighting people; it certainly felt as though he was at war, but in reality, he wasn't. He had been released from that situation twenty-nine years prior.

Are there things that seem or feel so true about God to you but seem to contradict what the Bible says about Him?

102. "Hiroo Onoda-obituary," *The Telegraph*, January 17, 2014, http://www.telegraph.co.uk/news/obituaries/10579800/Hiroo-Onoda-obituary.html?fb (accessed 29 May 2015).

On the surface this may seem like a strange question. But let me ask you: if Jesus appeared to you and went everywhere with you for twenty-four hours, would your behavior for that day change? How would you treat those you live with? How would you be in traffic? How would you relate to those who are homeless, who ask you for food? I suspect your behavior would change. I am sure mine would. However, Jesus specifically promised to us that He, and the Father, would come and make their home in us.[103] If God has promised that He is with us always,[104] then why, sometimes, do we live as if it isn't true?

The reason this happens, says New York pastor Tim Keller, is that we develop what he calls "defeater beliefs."[105] Defeater beliefs are things we believe about life that make it difficult for some of the truth we read in the Bible to seem or feel true to us. For instance, there may be times in our life when we have cried out to God, and He has seemed far away. In the perceived pain of not being answered, a defeater belief may have developed in our hearts that God isn't always with us. So when we read verses like, *"I will never leave you or forsake you"* (Hebrews 13:5), because of this defeater belief the verse doesn't transfer from "head" knowledge to "heart" knowledge. In other words, we tell people it is true but live as if it isn't.

We develop defeater beliefs without realizing it. They can develop in response to a specific emotional experience, such as a parent or teacher speaking negative words over us, or they can develop gradually, a little bit at a time, as we listen to the views of the friends we hang around with, to the books we read, or to the movies or TV shows we watch.

When I was going through my teenage years, the sitcom *Friends* was at the height of its popularity. I really enjoyed the

---

103. See John 14:23.
104. See Matthew 28:20.
105. See Tim Keller, *Deconstructing Defeater Beliefs: Leading the Secular to Christ*, www.welcometoredeemer.com/s/Apologetics_and_Outreach.pdf (accessed 29 May 2015).

humor and friendship that was modeled in the show, but it also coincided with the period of my life when my friendship with God was strained. After watching one particular show I remember thinking, "Have I chosen well? Sex is portrayed so casually, and as so little of a deal, has God got it right for me to abstain from sex until marriage?" A defeater belief was trying to creep in to my heart that said, "God's sexual ethic can't be right because everyone around me seems to be living by a different ethic, and they seem much happier than me. Surely, if God's ethic was true, I wouldn't be this unhappy about it!"

If attractive lifestyles in the media or Hollywood can generate defeater beliefs, on the opposite side negative experiences, particularly traumatic ones, are also powerful generators of defeater beliefs: "God can't be both loving and powerful, if He let _____ happen to me!" or "Where was God when _____ took place? It can't be true that even when we walk through death's valley He is there with us."

Although these words in the Bible are true, they often don't seem or feel true because of our negative experiences. The culture we grow up in, the people we are influenced by, and the experiences we have all had shape our heart beliefs. Have you ever heard people reject things out of hand without thinking too much about it? They might say something like, "That doesn't seem true" or "No, that just doesn't feel right." When beliefs get into our heart they determine what we view and feel to be normal. When something new comes along it either fits into our belief pattern, where we readily accept it, or it is in opposition to our belief pattern, and we usually automatically reject it. Occasionally a third thing happens, and we are so struck by the new concept that we absorb it and let it adjust the beliefs in our heart.

This is why the Bible will always challenge our beliefs. No matter how much we enjoy the culture we were brought up in, no culture is entirely lined up with the biblical worldview. For instance, those of us from a Western culture will resonate with the Bible when it tells us that God is love. That's what we'd expect God to be, but those from a Middle Eastern culture often find this concept something to grapple with. In contrast, a lot of Westerners grapple with the out-workings of the justice of God, but Middle Eastern Christians often find this quite intuitive—it just seems true that God is just in condemning people who disobey him.

As Christians, our responsibility is to allow God's truth, not our culture or our inclinations, to be the thing that adjusts the beliefs in our hearts, so that our heart increasingly lines up with God's heart. In other words, we must continually allow any defeater beliefs present in our heart to be replaced with God's truth.

HOW THIS AFFECTS HEALING

It is important to ensure we believe the truth about God in the area of healing because false beliefs could stop us from accessing any healing He wants to offer us. For example, what would have happened if the Roman centurion with the sick servant didn't really believe that Jesus had authority over sickness?[106] He may not have approached Jesus for healing, and his servant may have died. What would have happened if the Syrophoenician woman wasn't sure that Jesus was merciful and compassionate?[107] After being initially refused healing, maybe she wouldn't have persisted in asking for deliverance for her daughter.

What if the others at the Pool of Bethesda had discovered the truth that the Creator of the universe was standing in front of them?[108] Maybe they would have called out for healing from Jesus, instead of putting their hope in a rumored angelic visitation.

If you remember some of the incidents from chapter 1, we could also ask similar questions. What if Amy had rejected my

---

106. See Luke 7:2–10.
107. See Mark 7:24–30.
108. See John 5:1–9.

thought that she could have a toxic goiter? Or what if Hannah hadn't believed that God operates in physical healing today? What would have happened if the mother of the boy who was dumb didn't believe that Jesus had something to offer her son, after the doctors couldn't help?

Truth matters. And truth that we keep in our heart about God matters the most.

TRUTH AND THE TRINITY[109]

God has revealed Himself to us as one God in three Persons. Each Person of the Trinity is equal in value and worth, and because of what Jesus has done, we get the opportunity to interact with each of them. However, if you asked various people if there is a member of the Trinity they find themselves interacting with more, you'll often find that people do have a preference, and interestingly, which member of the Trinity this is varies from person to person. Some people will find themselves commonly addressing God the Father, while others will direct their prayers to Jesus more. Others still will find it easiest to pray to the Holy Spirit.

Counseling experience has shown this preference is often linked to good and bad role models in our life growing up. For example, if a close friend betrayed us, it becomes harder to respond to the friendship Jesus offers us. On the other hand, if we had a warm, affirming father who always protected and provided for us, it is often easier to relate to God revealed to us as Father. Because one of the roles of the Holy Spirit is to be our Teacher, good or bad experiences from those who taught us will make it easier or harder to connect to the Holy Spirit in this way.

At the end of the chapter I'll take you through a process that allows you to identify any defeater beliefs you may have, ask God to remove

---

109. This section is based on the teaching of Teresa Liebscher and Dawn da Silva, Bethel Church, Redding, California, who developed this concept as part of their inner healing process, *Bethel Sozo*.

them, and then replace them with His truth, but before that I want to look at each member of the Trinity and their biblically revealed roles, and outline common defeater beliefs that develop around them.

GOD THE FATHER

Jesus said He came to show us the Father.[110] In the New Testament Jesus and His disciples refer to God as Father over one hundred and fifty times. In doing this, Jesus wasn't referring to a passive, distant Father. He often used the Aramaic word abba, which is an intimate word for "father" that is still used in Israel today. I heard somebody who had travelled to Israel relate how he had seen a father and a young son holding hands while walking down the street. When the boy saw a toy in a shop window he jumped up and down, excitedly shouting, "Abba, abba!" or "Daddy, daddy!" In using the word abba so frequently, Jesus was changing the Jewish mind-set from one of God as almighty but a little distant, to one of a God who is deeply personal. In the Lord's Prayer, Jesus teaches us to pray, *"Our Father"* (Matthew 6:9). Jesus' aim was that we should have this same, deep connection with God the Father that He had. There were three key areas that the Father was particularly active in Jesus' life: identity/value, provision, and protection.

Mary's Story

During a time of prayer Mary asked the Holy Spirit to reveal how she saw God the Father. In her mind she saw a picture of somebody far off and distant. Her earthly father had been emotionally distant, so she forgave him for this. She then went on to say sorry to God for believing that He, as God the Father, was similar to this. As she repented of believing this lie, the picture in her mind changed dramatically, and she sensed that God the Father was very close to her. It now felt true that God the Father was somebody she could go to for affirmation.

110. See John 14:8–11.

Identity and Value

At Jesus' baptism, and then later on the Mount of Transfiguration, we see God the Father publicly affirming Jesus, saying, *"You are my Son, whom I love; with you I am well pleased"* (Luke 3:22 NIV). Jesus didn't need to look to success or human affirmation to give Him His worth or sense of value. Instead, He got this from His Father in heaven. When the crowds threatened to kill Him, and some of His disciples left Him, He remained secure that He was in the Father's will.[111] He knew He was loved by His Father and this enabled Him to freely love others. Thus He could confidently say, *"As the Father has loved me, so have I loved you"* (John 15:9).

As well as value, God the Father also gave Jesus a strong sense of identity. Jesus wasn't shaken when the religious leaders said He was working for a demonic prince, because His Father in heaven had confirmed who He was really representing.[112]

Good fathers follow God in this. They instill in us a sense of identity and worth. A pastor I know, PJ Smyth, felt very strongly about the role a father has instilling identity in children. When his children complained that their friends weren't held to the same standards they were, he would regularly say to them, "But you are Smyth boys; your friends aren't. They may do things differently, but this is what we Smyths do."

If our fathers do not model this aspect of God's character well—if they weren't around, if they were preoccupied, or if they were unsure of their identity themselves—then we may subconsciously reject God's ability to give us an identity. If this is the case, we can often spend our lives searching for identity in career, wealth, relationships, or anything that we think might do it. You can see this defeater belief in people who go from relationship to relationship, not able to be alone; needing somebody to always affirm their

---

111. See John 10:31; 6:66.
112. See Matthew 12:24.

beauty, worth, or importance. You see it also in people who drive themselves and others to be successful, as if it were a matter of life or death; sadly, if their identity is tied up in being a success, then being successful really will feel like a matter of life or death to them!

Dale's Story

Dale's parents were intravenous drug users, and so at birth he was put up for adoption. Dale's adopted dad loved him very much but was both a strict disciplinarian and emotionally reserved, and Dale didn't feel close to him. Dale was very troubled during his teenage years, was drawn into practicing the occult, and became addicted to drugs. On becoming a Christian he received prayer ministry and was freed of his drug addiction. Things went well for a while, and Dale got married, but when his marriage hit a rocky patch, he went back to drugs. He came to see me during this crisis and because of his experiences growing up, he realized that he found it very difficult to connect to God as Father; consequently, he struggled with a lot of fear. During a time of prayer he forgave his biological dad for rejecting him and his adoptive dad for not fully modeling God's Fatherly heart to him. He renounced the lie that God the Father didn't want to be emotionally close to him, and he was able to be free of the fear that had gripped him. Because of this new connection to God the Father, he was able to reconcile with his wife, and they are together to this day.

In contrast, God wants to give us a different measure of success, and He wants to be the One who gives us our identity and sense of worth, so that we don't have to seek for it in created things. When you become born again, any failure by your earthly father to instill the right sense of value and identity in you no longer needs to be a hindrance in life. God the Father can fill any gap left by father figures. However, the way for this to happen is to first deal with any defeater beliefs that may have crept in.

How are you doing in this area? If you are a believer, can you find your identity and value in being a child of God or do you tend to look to created things to give you a sense of value or self-worth?

Provision

During Jesus' three years of ministry He travelled around Israel without knowing where He would sleep or where His meals would come from, yet He was never in lack. For example, when He needed a place to have His last supper, His Father provided the perfect place for Him.[113] When He needed an animal to enter Jerusalem, in line with the prophecies about Him, His Father revealed to Him where His disciples would find one.[114]

Nowadays, in most families, both parents tend to go out to work at some point in their lives, but God holds the father of the family responsible to ensure there is enough for his family.[115] If our fathers, or those who took the place of fathers, do not model this aspect of God's character, a defeater belief is often created that God won't provide for us. When this belief is present, it can makes us put too much value on wealth and the security that accumulating wealth can bring. During good times we'll be at peace, but during difficult times, if reserves are low, we'll be prone to experience a lot of anxiety.

Protection

Jesus was very aware of the protection His father offered, because even as He was about to be arrested in the garden of Gethsemane, He said to Peter, *"Do you think that I cannot appeal to my Father, and he will at once send me more than twelve legions of angels?"* (Matthew 26:53).[116]

---

113. See Mark 14:13–16.
114. See Mark 11:2–6.
115. See 1 Timothy 5:8.
116. About 60,000 angels (the standard Roman legion was typically 4500–5500 men).

Children should feel safe and protected by fathers. Children love to boast in this feeling. Maybe you heard the common playground chant, "My Dad's bigger than your Dad"? It is a boast in how protected child feel by their fathers. Fathers often feel a special sense of duty to protect when they have daughters and, symbolically, when a daughter gets married, it is the father who hands her over to her husband to symbolize that the husband is taking over the duty of protection.

If fathers do not model this sense of protection well, people often find it hard to know God the Father as their protector. They may develop a lot of fear or try and take control of their safety, for example, by anxiously learning martial arts, or, through worry, always having a weapon close by. They may also have an overly strong desire to live in safer areas, or make other decisions about career or family choices on the basis of safety. While some caution is wise, God the Father wants us to be able to trust Him in this area and receive wisdom for safety from Him.

GOD THE SON

When we were adopted into God's family, we gained Jesus as an older brother. It is Jesus who models to us what it is like to live as God's child, but additionally, He is accessible to us in the same way a close sibling or good friend should be. Jesus demonstrated this while on earth through the close, brothering relationships He had with His disciples. They travelled together, ate together, and shared experiences together. They went through trying times, but they also had a lot of fun; Jesus even created nicknames for some of them![117]

Jesus offers that same relationship to us. However, because of the development of defeater beliefs, our ability to access this type of relationship is shaped by our relationships with earthly siblings

---

117. Simon was called *kêpâ*, literally "stone" in Aramaic, which developed into Cephas or Peter. James and John were called *Boanerges*, Aramaic for the "Sons of Thunder," and Thomas was nicknamed *tômâ*, Aramaic for "twin."

or close friends. Here are some of the elements of a sibling relationship that Jesus modeled to us.

Paulo's Story

Paulo became a Christian in his early twenties and would tell everyone about God. As time went on, his passion cooled. One thing that he could never really understand was the idea that he could relate to Jesus in the same way that he would with his close friends. Growing up, Paulo was often lonely as a child because his siblings were between ten to twenty years older than him, and he was bullied at school. Forgiving his older siblings for not being interested in him as a child enabled him to renounce the lie that Jesus would be as his siblings were to him. His view of Jesus changed and he could relate a lot better to Him after the prayer time.

Friendship

Jesus said to His disciples, *"No longer do I call you servants... but I have called you friends, for all I have heard from my Father I have made known to you"* (John 15:15), and *"To you it has been given to know the secrets of the kingdom"* (Matthew 13:11). Some people are best friends with their siblings, knowing each other's deepest secrets; others fell out with their siblings a long time ago and don't even talk to them anymore. How our siblings relate to us in the realm of friendship often filters how we see the friendship Jesus offers us.

Discipleship

During our childhood years, our parents answer many of our questions about life, but as we grow older we look to our peers and (if we have them) older siblings to teach us. We often get "discipled" in their ways of doing things, and our experience of life is deeply affected by them. Jesus guided His disciples through formal teaching, through modeling, and through sending them out and getting them to report back. By so doing, the disciples trusted Jesus and learned His ways.

If our siblings are cold toward us, needy, overbearing, or break our trust, these may create defeater beliefs about brotherly friendship, and it can be difficult to connect to Jesus as our Discipler. People who have this block often understand Jesus as their Savior, but do not have a close, everyday experience of discipleship with Him or submission to His ways.

Mike's Story

Mike grew up in a traditional church, but it was a very minor part of his life. His faith only became real when he started going to an evangelical church in his late teens. However, he found the concept of the Holy Spirit being a Person rather than a force very difficult to grasp. Through prayer he realized that his parents hadn't been good at comforting and nurturing him as a young child. In particular he realized his mother had quite a controlling tendency that kept him from wanting to share life's problems with her. In the past, when he had shared, he often felt coerced into doing things that he didn't like. During a time of prayer he was able forgive his parents and say sorry to God for not believing the truth in his heart that God could be his Comforter and Counselor.

GOD THE HOLY SPIRIT

Jesus said it would be better for us if He were to go to heaven and send the Holy Spirit to us rather than stay on the earth in person.[118] If we remember the impact Jesus' presence made on the disciple's lives, that's quite a statement about the Spirit's power!

---

118. See John 16:7.

The Holy Spirit has many roles. He is there to convict us of sin and guide us in truth, allowing God's Word to enter our hearts.[119] He is the Giver of gifts and the Source of spiritual fruit.[120] In John 14–16, Jesus explained that the Holy Spirit would be sent to be our Counselor, Comforter, and Teacher.[121]

Some Christians have a close relationship with the Holy Spirit, while others find it harder to connect to Him. Defeater beliefs develop about Holy Spirit when those who model the Spirit's roles do so in a way that is deficient. I have found a lot of defeater beliefs have developed in people around the roles of the Holy Spirit of counselor, comforter, and teacher and would like to look at these in more detail.

Counselor

If we found it difficult to go to our parents for advice we may find it difficult to see the Holy Spirit as a Person to get advice and counsel from. But Jesus specifically sent the Holy Spirit to fulfill that role for us. If we identify the defeater belief, we can remove this block and allow the Holy Spirit to be our first port of call for counsel.

Comforter

When the early church had gone through persecution, it had a season of restoration. During this time, Luke tells us that all the churches in Judea, Galilee, and Samaria walked in the *comfort of the Holy Spirit*" (Acts 9:31). Jesus sent the Holy Spirit to us when He went to heaven, and during times of difficulty the Holy Spirit can similarly bring us comfort. When we are children, the person who comforts us is usually our mother, but in some situations it is another relative or a nanny. In modern Western families the father has a greater role in comforting than previous eras. Our experience

---

119. See John 16:8, 13.
120. See 1 Corinthians 12:11; Galatians 5:22–23.
121. See especially John 14:26.

of these comforting relationships affects how we see the Holy Spirit as Comforter. If we lacked comfort in our home growing up, it can be difficult to see the Holy Spirit as able to offer comfort either. When we need comfort, then, we may easily go elsewhere. The reason people depend on external things for comfort (such as alcohol, shopping, eating, etc.) in times of stress is because there is often a defeater belief present that stops them from approaching God for comfort.

Teacher

The Holy Spirit is promised to guide us *"into all the truth"* (John 16:13). If we had good teachers (initially parents, and later, school teachers) who made us feel safe to ask questions and inquire, then we will probably find it easy understand truth from the Holy Spirit. However, if we were made to feel stupid or that our questions were an annoyance, then there may be a heart-level defeater belief present that is stopping us from approaching the Holy Spirit as our Teacher.

PRACTICAL STEPS *TO REMOVE DEFEATER BELIEFS*

For biblical truth to be implanted in our hearts, we need to first repent of any defeater beliefs that we have developed that may be in opposition to that particular truth. Alongside this, we need to forgive those people who created the situation that allowed a defeater belief to develop.

I have found it helpful to forgive people for this, even if those people were unaware they were doing this. To keep things brief, instead of using the phrase "saying you're sorry for developing defeater beliefs" I'll just use the word *renounce*. For example, you might sense that you are believing a defeater belief that God isn't emotionally close. I simply suggest you to declare: "I renounce the lie that God is emotionally distant from me, and I forgive _____ for modeling this to me."

STEP A: SETTING THE SCENE

+ Choose a place where you won't be disturbed.

+ Choose a moment when you will not be interrupted.

+ Turn off your cell phone.

+ Grab a pen, paper, and a willing heart to respond to God.

+ If you feel it would be helpful, ask a trusted Christian friend to be with you and quietly pray as you go through the process.

STEP B: GOD THE FATHER

+ Write down the main people (if more than one) who have taken on a fathering role in your life.

+ Write down anybody whom you feel should have had a fathering role in your life, but didn't (e.g. an absent biological father, a stepfather who didn't take an active interest, etc.)

1. Identity & Value

a) Does it seem true or feel true that God the Father deeply values you?

Yes / Mostly / Sometimes / Not at all

If you answered anything other than yes, declare out loud: "I renounce the lie that God the Father doesn't value me or that He is emotionally distant." Using the principles from chapter 5, forgive anybody on the two lists above who did not fully model God's character to you in this area.

b) Does it seem true or feel true that if all your other roles (parent, spouse, child, brother/sister, role at work) and successes in life were taken away, being a child of God would be enough?

Yes / Mostly / Sometimes / Not at all

If you answered anything other than yes, declare out loud: "I renounce the lie that God the Father is not able to or doesn't want to give me an identity based in Him." Using the principles from chapter 5, forgive anybody on the lists above for not fully modeling God's heart toward you in this area.

2. Provision

a) Does it seem true or feel true that God the Father is able to provide for your needs?

Yes / Mostly / Sometimes / Not at all

If you answered anything other than yes, declare out loud: "I renounce the lie that God the Father is not able to or doesn't want to provide for my needs." Again, using the principles from chapter 5, forgive anybody on the lists above for not fully modeling God's heart toward you in this area.

3. Protection

a) Does it seem true or feel true that God the Father is able to be your Protector?

Yes / Mostly / Sometimes / Not at all

If you answered anything other than yes, declare out loud: "As His child, I renounce the lie that God the Father is not able to or doesn't want to protect me." Using the principles from chapter 5, forgive anybody on the lists above for not fully modeling God's heart toward you.

STEP C: GOD THE SON

+ Write down the names of your siblings (include half-brothers/sisters, step-brother/sisters), and anybody who has seemed as close to you as a sibling.

1. Friendship

Does it seem true or feel true that you can speak to Jesus as you would a close friend?

Yes / Mostly / Sometimes / Not at all

If you answered anything other than yes, declare out loud: "I renounce the lie that Jesus does not want to or is not able to have a close friendship with me." Using the principles from chapter 5, forgive anybody on the lists above for not fully modeling the brotherly friendship that Jesus offers you.

2. Discipleship

Does it seem true or feel true that you are able to go to Jesus to learn about everyday life and that He is willing to help you follow in His footsteps?

Yes / Mostly / Sometimes / Not at all

If you answered anything other than yes, declare out loud: "I renounce the lie that Jesus is not able to or doesn't want to guide me through everyday life." Using the principles from chapter 5, forgive anybody on the lists above (or others) for not fully modeling the ability to guide, coach, or disciple you.

STEP D: GOD THE HOLY SPIRIT

+ Write down the main people (if more than one) who have taken on a comforting/counseling role in your life.

+ Write down anybody who you feel should have been there to comfort or counsel you, but, for whatever reason, didn't (e.g. an absent biological mother/father, a distant stepmother or father, etc.).

1. Comforter

a) When you feel stressed or distressed, is the Holy Spirit the first place you go to for comfort?

Yes / Mostly / Sometimes / Not at all

If you answered anything other than yes, declare out loud: "I renounce the lie that the Holy Spirit isn't a person I can go to in order to receive comfort." Using the principles from chapter 5, forgive anybody on the lists above for not fully modeling God's heart toward you in this area.

2. Counselor

a) Does it seem true or feel true that the Holy Spirit is a good source of advice and help to you?

Yes / Mostly / Sometimes / Not at all

If you answered anything other than yes, declare out loud: "I renounce the lie that the Holy Spirit isn't a Person I can go to in order to receive comfort." Using the principles from chapter 5, forgive anybody on the lists above for not fully modeling God's heart toward you in this area.

3. Teacher

a) Does it seem true or feel true that the Holy Spirit is able and available to teach you all that you need to know?

Yes / Mostly / Sometimes / Not at all

If you answered anything other than yes, declare out loud: "I renounce the lie that the Holy Spirit isn't a Person I can go to in order to receive teaching." Using the principles from chapter 5, forgive anybody on the lists above for not fully modeling God's heart toward you in this area.

KEY POINTS

1. Through our experiences in life, we can subconsciously take on false beliefs that may seem or feel true but actually are not.

2. If we develop false beliefs about God, they can hinder us from fully coming to Him for healing.

3. False beliefs about God can be removed through turning away from them and forgiving the people that may have actively or passively participated in creating them.

CHAPTER 7:

REORDERING LOVE?

"Pride costs us more than hunger, thirst, and cold."
—*Thomas Jefferson*
Third President of the United States

At the turn of the millennium, the music industry was in crisis. People stopped purchasing music from shops and instead began to swap it digitally between their friends and anyone on the net who was willing. A major source of income for the industry had been royalties from purchases, but that income rapidly dropped as it became increasingly acceptable to not pay for music. The big five players in the market were divided on how to proceed and were facing a downturn. But out of the blue came Steve Jobs with his rejuvenated company, Apple, and he gifted them a complete solution: Apple's brand-new iTunes store would sell songs online so that people could download them onto their beautifully designed portable music device, the iPod. The rest, as they say, is history.

Some CEOs may possibly turn an industry upside down in their lifetime, but Jobs went on to not only save the music industry, but to also rejuvenate the flagging cell phone market with the revolutionary iPhone. Through his other company, Pixar, he transformed animated movies. He also introduced us to the computer mouse, colorful graphics, and more recently, to the iPhone and the iPad. In 2009, Fortune magazine named him CEO of the Decade and, in 2012, declared him to be the "the greatest entrepreneur of our time." For a brief period, Apple, the company he co-founded in his parents' garage, became the most valuable company in the world.

This entrepreneurial brilliance came to an abrupt end when, in October 2011, at the age of fifty-six, he passed away from a rare pancreatic tumor. Sadly, if it wasn't for self-confessed stubbornness and pride on his part, this early death may have been entirely prevented.

Jobs was diagnosed with a glucagonoma, a rare cancer of that develops from the islet cells of the pancreas.[122] Only one in twenty million people ever get this cancer. Fifty percent of the time it is detected late, having already spread to other parts of the body, and death is only a short time away. However, if it is detected prior to spreading, there is a good chance that it can be removed surgically and the patient survive.

In Jobs' case, by a stroke of luck, his cancer was detected early, in 2003. A chance encounter with one of his doctors led to him having a follow-up scan on his kidneys. His kidneys were clear of the stones he had suffered from a few years earlier, but the scan picked up something unusual in the pancreas. His urologist urged him to get it checked out, but Jobs wasn't keen. After her persistence, he agreed to have a biopsy taken, which revealed the glucagonoma. Most people, on discovering cancer in their body, would want it removed immediately but, to the horror of his close friends and family, he refused, saying to his biographer later, with some regret, "I really didn't want them to open up my body, so I tried to see if a few other things would work."[123]

---

122. See http://emedicine.medscape.com/article/118899-overview#a0199.
123. W. Isaacson, *Steve Jobs* (New York: Simon & Schuster, 2011), 454.

The "few other things" included massive quantities of blended fruit and carrot juice, acupuncture, herbal remedies, hydrotherapy, and a talking therapy where he was encouraged to express all his negative emotion. Nine months later, with friendships at near breaking points, he agreed to have a rescan and discovered, to his horror, that the cancer had not only grown, but had spread.

During the next eight years Jobs used his wealth to fight the cancer with the best technology and medication there was. He spent over one hundred thousand dollars to get his genome sequenced (a computerized record of all his DNA), enabling his doctors to select the drugs that were most suited to him and his cancer's genetic make-up. He travelled to Switzerland for experimental treatment, but his health continued to decline. After having a liver transplant in 2009, he continued to deteriorate, passing away two years later from progression of the disease.

Nobody really knows whether, if he had listened to his friends, family, and doctors when the cancer was first detected, he'd be still around alive today. Some say that with his particular cancer, it wouldn't have mattered, but personally I suspect there would have been a good chance. At the very least, having the surgery before the cancer had spread would have been a much better starting point to fight it from, rather than first trying alternative medicines.

Pride has a huge effect on health. It was because of King Nebuchadnezzar's pride that God arranged for him to experience seven years of madness.[124] It was only when he acknowledged that God was God, and that he wasn't, that God allowed him to regain his sanity. Namaan, the ancient Syrian army commander, nearly didn't get healed of his leprous skin disease because he thought God's instruction for healing was too simple and a bit demeaning.[125] Pharaoh's pride in not submitting to God led him and his people to experience the twelve plagues, of which three were

---

124. See Daniel 4:4–37.
125. See 2 Kings 5:1–14.

directly sicknesses.[126] King David's pride in wanting to know the exact strength of his army caused him to skip over God's requirements for taking a census, resulting in a disease that caused seventy thousand deaths.[127]

The apostle James sums it up quite bluntly, saying that God *"opposes the proud"* (James 4:6). You can probably cope with many opponents in life, but if there is one being you don't want to be in opposition to, it is God.

WHAT IS PRIDE?

If pride is so destructive to our physical and spiritual health, it is important we understand exactly what it is, so that we can avoid it. Pride is a confusing word because although it is predominantly used negatively,[128] it is sometimes used positively as well.[129] Pride can manifest itself in hundreds of ways—pride in our appearance, our work, our family, or our country, to name just a few. The church father Augustine assigned it a morally neutral status, simply calling it the "love of one's own excellence." However, pride may not be that neutral; the overarching use of pride in Scripture is negative. When the world-renowned preacher and writer, John Piper, announced an eight-month leave of absence in order to deal with "several species of pride in my soul"[130] it wasn't something positive, but something that was harming his ministry. The Bible tells us that *"Pride goes before destruction, and a haughty spirit before a fall"* (Proverbs 16:18). It is worth taking note that Piper saw that it was better to be proactive and deal with pride than suffer from its effects.

---

126. See Exodus 5–12.
127. See 1 Chronicles 21:1–14.
128. See Ezekiel 28:17; Jeremiah 13:15; 1 Peter 5:5; and James 4:6.
129. See 2 Corinthians 7:4; 1 Corinthians 15:31.
130. John Piper, "Upcoming Leave," DesiringGod.com, April 21, 2015, www. desiringgod.org/articles/john-pipers-upcoming-leave (accessed 23 April 2015).

Thomas Aquinas, the fourteenth-century Italian theologian, gave us a more specific definition of the bad form of pride: "inordinate self-love and the cause of every sin…it is refusing to be subject to God and His rule." Self-love doesn't sound so bad, you may think. Jesus told us we are to love our neighbor as we love our self.[131] But Thomas Aquinas doesn't tell us that pride is self-love. He says that pride is an *inordinate* (excessive or disproportionately large) amount of self-love; such an amount that it blocks us from submitting to God and His rule. Effectively, excessive self-love causes us to commit cosmic treason and replace ourselves as ruler of our lives, instead of God.

It can happen gradually but can also reach a crisis. A friend of mind said to me once: "I am not sure I like Christianity because to do it properly there is too big a cost. I mean, if I allow Jesus to be Lord then He may send me to Outer Mongolia, and I have plans for my life and they don't include going to Outer Mongolia!" While my friend had misunderstood God's heart (what He asks of us is always, ultimately best for us), he correctly understood the tension between self-love and love for God. Sadly for my friend, he turned his back on his church upbringing and his experience of God, and self-love won.

Excessive love of self is easy to spot in others, but it is often harder to spot in ourselves. We are often not as honest with ourselves as my friend was, but all of us are likely to be teetering on the brink of our self-love being greater than our love for God, as this joke points to: A man was once late for a meeting but he couldn't find anywhere to park his car, so in desperation he prayed to God and said, "God, if you help me find a parking spot I'll promise to go to church every Sunday for a whole year." Just as he was finishing praying a parking spot opened up right in front of him, and he quickly added, "Actually, no need to bother, God. I've found one myself!"

---

131. See Matthew 22:39.

Stephen Fry on Self-Pity

The British comedic actor Stephen Fry, as a long-term sufferer from bipolar disorder, knows the dangers of self-pity all too well. He describes it this way: "Self-pity will destroy relationships, it'll destroy anything that's good, it will fulfill all the prophecies it makes and leave only itself. And it's so simple to imagine that one is hard done by, and that things are unfair, and that one is underappreciated, and that if only one had had a chance at this, only one had had a chance at that, things would have gone better, you would be happier if only this, that one is unlucky. All those things. And some of them may well even be true. But, to pity oneself as a result of them is to do oneself an enormous disservice."[132]

When our self-love overrides the love that we have for God, it should actually be described as self-worship. A friend of mine who was leading a church had on his team a number of young guys in their twenties. Once when they were holding a time of introspection, wanting to root out unhelpful practices, they took turns describing what they were struggling with. As the group questioned each other, almost without exception the root was traced back, with much shock, to self-worship, or pride.

Pride can be expressed in two main ways. We can feel superior to others, which is referred to as haughtiness or boasting, or we can feel inferior to others, which is referred to as self-pity. Both are forms of pride. In his book *What Jesus Demands from the World*, John Piper makes this helpful comparison:

Boasting is the response of pride to success. Self-pity is the response of pride to suffering. Boasting says, "I deserve admiration because I have achieved so much." Self-pity says, "I deserve admiration because I have sacrificed so

132. See https://www.youtube.com/watch?v=r_2kelqYz_o.

much." Boasting is the voice of pride in the heart of the strong. Self-pity is the voice of pride in the heart of the weak. Boasting sounds self-sufficient. Self-pity sounds self-sacrificing. The reason self-pity does not look like pride is that it appears to be so needy. But the need arises from a wounded ego. It doesn't come from a sense of unworthiness, but from a sense of unrecognized worthiness. It is the response of unapplauded pride.[133]

C. S. Lewis says that pride is simply the "ruthless, sleepless, unsmiling concentration upon self." Unsmiling, because when we can laugh at ourselves we are aware of our faults, but when we cannot laugh, it is because we don't want to be seen to have faults. Which form of self-focus do you tend toward? Boasting or self-pity? Or maybe, like me, you have times when both apply? If you have been sick for a long time, self-pity can often be a very real temptation. If you have gloried in your own achievements or shunned other people's input, as Steve Jobs discovered, sickness may be something that catches up with you.

WHAT IS ANGER?

"Anybody can become angry—that is easy, but to be angry with the right person, to the right degree, at the right time, for the right purpose, and in the right way—that is not easy!"
—*Aristotle*

Pride usually manifests itself, sooner or later, in anger because when our pride collides with the recalcitrant reality of life, anger is usually the reaction. It's the more visible child of arrogance; even when people can't see your pride, they can see your anger.

---

133. John Piper, *Desiring God: Meditations of a Christian Hedonist* (Sisters, OR: Multnomah, 2003), 302.

Anger poses no small threat to our health. The author Mark Twain said, "Anger is an acid that can do more harm to the vessel in which it is stored than to anything in which it is poured." Science has shown that Mark Twain's analogy is nearer the truth than he probably realized. Anger is now associated with increased risk of stomach ulcers, high blood pressure, and coronary heart disease. Retained anger really does corrode our insides. One scientific study showed the biological link between anger and coronary heart disease by demonstrating that people with high levels of hostility had increased levels of Tumour Necrosis Factor Alpha (TNFa), one of the PICs we mentioned in chapter 3.[134] In many heart diseases, TNFa, along with other PICs, attack the wall of the coronary arteries and cause cholesterol to attach to the passageway. This build-up causes the artery to become narrower and narrower until eventually it is completely blocked off. Without blood flow to that part of the heart, the heart tissue dies, which is why a heart attack is so painful—part of your heart is dying. If you get treatment quickly enough, you can prevent the tissue death, but in many cases people do not, and they are left with dead tissue in that part of the heart.

I spent three months working on a coronary heart ward, with people who had just had heart attacks. In some of the people, you could almost see the anger they were carrying. Anger is an emotion, but as Tim Keller explained, anger is not just something you *feel*, but something you *do*.[135] You get angry. Your fists clench, your heart speeds up, the veins around your head fill up with blood, your face scowls. With some people I meet, I can see the effects that regular anger has on them. Their whole countenance seems to give off hostility, and they develop anger lines and tensed muscles.

134. E. C. Suarez et al., "The relation of aggression, hostility, and anger to lipopolysaccharide-stimulated tumor necrosis factor (TNF)-alpha by blood monocytes from normal men," *Brain Behavior and Immunity* 16, no. 6 (December 2002): 675–84.

135. Tim Keller, "The Healing of Anger," sermon preached 17 October 2004, Redeemer Presbyterian Church, New York, http://sermons2.redeemer.com/sermons/healing-anger (accessed 29 May 2015).

Tim Keller goes on to refer to anger as "dynamite of the soul." With some angry people, you have to be quite careful around them in case the dynamite goes off and you get caught in the explosion.

You might not be the explosive type, but all of us can relate to anger at some level. Dr. Henry Brandt, a medical missionary to Africa, made this candid assessment:

> Not everyone is an alcoholic; not everyone steals, or swears, or commits adultery. But everyone struggles with anger. It is a universal problem. I have observed it among primitive cannibals in Irian Jaya, among illiterate people in tiny villages deep in the forest of Zaire, among my play-mates when I was a child, in my parents, in church members, in pastors, in highly educated people, in the very rich, in people in government. And yes, in me.[136]

During my three months' stay in Ghana, I saw a vivid example of how anger can give a foothold to evil. Culturally, Ghana has embraced Christianity more than any nation I have come across. For instance, the local bakery was called "Jesus is the bread of life" and it wouldn't be unusual to come across the "Jesus will wash you clean" launderette. It was a deeply spiritual place but also very dualistic. I saw a taxi with the sticker "Jesus saves" next a sticker for *Playboy* magazine. People would go to a local pastor for prayer for healing, but then go visit the local witch doctor, as well. I remember asking one of the medical students how they dealt with people going to witch doctors before coming to the hospital. She casually replied, "Everybody believes in evil spirits; you grow up around them." Ghanaians understood that witch doctors had one way of dealing with them and Christianity had another.

It was after being invited to a local prayer field by one of the Christian medical students that I saw the effects of evil spirits first-hand. Each evening, the field was full of small groups of people

---

136. H. Brandt, "How to deal with anger," *Journal of Biblical Counseling* 16, no. 1 (Fall 1997): 28.

standing in circles singing, praying, or being preached at. I later found out these were small churches. One of the pastors befriended me and invited me to join his small church meetings. It turned out that he had quite a gift of discernment, and he told me he could see evil spirits that were connected to people. This may seem quite strange if you have grown up in a Western environment, but this is not uncommon in other parts of the world. It seems that, in a culture full of witchcraft and evil spirits, people had joined the church in hope that the pastor could use his spiritual gifts to protect them.

I was granted permission to follow up with those who were identified, and so I chatted with one of the ladies and asked God for the cause of her spiritual issue. I got the sense that anger was a problem in her life and so, remembering the proverb quoted in Ephesians, I asked if she had ever gone to bed angry and woken up still angry.[137] "Yes!" she replied with a lot of venom, "with my husband. He makes me very angry." I explained the Scripture to her and led her through forgiving her husband and repenting of her retained anger. I then prayed with her and asked the Holy Spirit to fill her. Instead of a demonic reaction, this time she experienced a lot of joy, and at the meetings she no longer reacted the way she had previously. I checked with the pastor who had the gift of discernment, and he told me he no longer saw a demon attached to her. By retaining anger, this lady had opened herself up to demonic oppression, but by confessing the anger and forgiving her husband, she was able to be set free.

Anger is not just universal but also addictive, and like any addictive substance, if we let it, it can control us. Proverbs warns of the danger of getting ensnared by anger if we make friends with angry people and goes on to say that we shouldn't rescue angry people from the results of their anger, otherwise we will have to rescue them again and again.[138] Given its bad health effects, both spiritually and physically, anger is something that we don't want to get ensnared by.

137. Ephesians 4:26
138. See Proverbs 22:24; 19:19.

Is all anger harmful? The daughter of the founding pastor of our church came running to him one day and said, "Dad, Dad, I have discovered something shocking! Jesus sinned!" He replied, "Really? Show me where you found this." She took him to the time when Jesus got angry in the temple courts.[139] He was able to turn the moment into a teaching session and explained that not all anger is sin, but if we do get angry our responsibility is to ensure we don't sin in our anger.[140]

As we saw in chapter 5, our emotions are morally neutral, and anger is no exception. What gives anger its moral component is determined by the motive. If our motive is selfish, theologians call the anger unrighteous anger, but if, like God, our motive is unselfish, then it is called righteous anger. This is a very important distinction because it is the sin component of anger that makes it so toxic. Unrighteous anger causes us to retain bitterness and live in unhealthy stress, but, conversely, righteous anger is actually healthy for us, as it energizes us to act for the sake of others, and it generates health-giving empathetic connections.

Righteous anger can be a cause for much good in the world. For instance, the anger William Wilberforce felt when he heard of the inhuman way slaves were being treated drove him to successfully call for slavery's abolition in the British Parliament. Anger at an injustice creates a healthy drive within us to overcome passivity and indifference. Instead of our anger being focused inward and used to destroy us, we point it outward at the injustice and use its destructive power for good. Consider also how Martin Luther King, Jr. channeled his anger to create passive resistance and peaceful civil rights marches to destroy racial segregation.

As well as being "dynamite of the soul," Tim Keller also refers to anger as "love in motion." We get angry, he says, when something we love is threatened. For instance, parents will instantly feel anger when somebody threatens their son or daughter. This is because they love their child so much. More trivially, when my

139. See John 2:13–17.
140. See Ephesians 4:26.

niece almost poured water on my laptop, I was surprised to see how quickly I snapped at her, demonstrating a real love for my laptop—or at least a love of not wanting to spend time and money getting it fixed! Given this concept, we should be unsurprised to discover that a loving God has to be a God of anger. The renowned biblical counselor, David Powlison, says that God is actually the angriest Being mentioned in the Bible.[141]

If anger and love are so intimately linked, then the more that people love, the more they will get angry with anything that threatens the object of their love. God has clearly shown that we are the object of His love, and so it is only right that He should be angry with the sin that not only threatens to, but actually does, destroy us. If God did not have anger toward sin, it would signify that He didn't love us.

While God's anger is a pure, loving anger, our anger is most often impure and selfish. If we analyze our anger we will find that usually what roused our anger was a love of ourselves. Put simply, we get angry toward God and others because we don't get our own way. We are the object of our own love, and we use anger to try and destroy anything that blocks this self-love. This is a misuse of anger and it is not what God designed it for. And as we have seen, this inward-focused anger has a destructive effect on our bodies. If you are sick long-term, it is quite common to develop anger toward God or others. Tragically, this anger, when it is not processed properly, is the cause of much illness, and stops many people from properly approaching God for healing.

ORDERING PRIDE AND ANGER

So what must we do to correct these problems?

The bad form of pride and the bad form of anger are both the result of disordered love. The only way we are able to stop an

---

141. David Powlison is Executive Director of the Christian Counseling and Education Foundation (CCEF).

unhealthy love of our self is to find something or somebody more worthy and more wonderful to capture our affection. Nobody wants a God opposing them. If there is a Creator who not only created us but also rescued us, then none of us would want our love of self to be greater than our love for Him. So why is that the case so often? The question we need to ask ourselves is, "How do I take the focus off of myself and place it onto God—and keep it there?"

The first thing we need to do if we have unhealthy pride or anger is to acknowledge that things are not right. We need to see that down in our heart, our love is disordered—that we fall short of Jesus' command to love God with all of our heart. God doesn't just want our obedience or good works, although these are good things. Primarily He wants our affection, our love. It is what all of us want in any relationship. We don't want our spouses to serve us or tell us how obedient they have been; we want their love. When you are truly in love you naturally desire to serve, to complement, to sacrifice. Likewise, we don't want our interaction with our children to be based just on a list of rules; we want to connect with them relationally. Jesus died so that we could be adopted by a Father who loves us dearly, and He died so that He could have a bride,[142] a people that He cherishes and loves, in the same way that a good husband cherishes his wife. Jesus died to win our affection and He'll pursue us until He wins our hearts fully.

How would you describe your heart toward God currently? Are you allowing Him to pursue you or are you hardening your heart toward Him? Like any relationship, if we have discovered a pattern of selfishness that has harmed the relationship, the first thing we need to do is apologize and ask for forgiveness. If you are feeling convicted of this, why not do it now?

Once you have repented of a disordered love, the next step is to ask God to change your affections, and to restore Him as your first love. To help the process, let's look at pride and anger separately.

---

142. See Revelation 19:7–8.

PRACTICAL STEPS

STEP A: SETTING THE SCENE

+ Choose a place where you won't be disturbed.

+ Choose a moment when you will not be interrupted.

+ Turn off your cell phone.

+ If you feel it would be helpful, ask a trusted Christian friend to be with you and quietly pray as you go through the process.

STEP B: PRIDE

+ Superior Pride

"Do not think of yourself more highly than you ought, but rather think of yourself with sober judgment, in accordance with the faith God has distributed to each of you."

(Romans 12:3 NIV)

Check any of the following that apply to you:

❑ I find it easier to spot faults in others than in myself.

❑ I am often defensive when people give negative criticism or feedback.

❑ I often find myself offended by people.

❑ I have a stronger desire to do my will than God's will.

❑ I am more dependent upon my strengths and resources than God's.

❑ I sometimes consider myself more important than others.

❑ I have a tendency to think that I do not have needs.

❑ I feel that people regularly overlook my achievements.

❑ I find it difficult to connect with people who are poorer than me or are from a lower social status.

❏   I sometimes tell "white lies" to cover up mistakes.

❏   I find it hard to celebrate other people's successes when I haven't been successful.

❏   I get frustrated when conversations drift away from the topic I was interested in.

❏   I get really annoyed when I am asked to do belittling tasks.

❏   I find it hard to acknowledge there are areas in which others are better than me.

❏   I find it hard to listen to people.

❏   I prefer to find my own way rather than taking advice from others.

❏   I find it hard to follow other people's lead.

❏   I get frustrated when others have the final say.

❏   I rarely say sorry to people, and if I do, it takes me a while to do so.

❏   I find it difficult to admit that I was wrong.

❏   I often think I understand humility better than other people do.

All of the statements would suggest the presence of superior pride. The list is not exhaustive but, in general, the more boxes you checked, the greater the degree of superior pride. Take a moment to say a prayer of repentance to God for these things.

+ Inferior Pride

"No temptation has overtaken you that is not common to man." (1 Corinthians 10:3)

Check any of the following that apply to you:

❏   I regularly feel sorry for myself.

❏   I regularly have bouts of low self-esteem.

❑ I sometimes find myself being secretly pleased when certain people are unsuccessful.

❑ I tend to be more of a people-pleaser than a God-pleaser.

❑ I tend to get embarrassed when the spotlight is on me but secretly enjoy it.

❑ I often feel people do not recognize the times I have been victimized.

❑ I wish others would comfort me more.

❑ I find it difficult to think of things that I am grateful for.

❑ I find it hard to empathize with other people's problems.

❑ I sometimes find myself fishing for compliments from people.

❑ I am motivated to serve others for the appreciation that I get.

❑ If people don't thank me or affirm me for work that I have done, I feel deeply annoyed or down about it.

❑ I really enjoy it when people give me their attention.

All of the statements above would suggest the presence of inferior pride. Similar to the exercise on superior pride, the list is not exhaustive but, in general, the more boxes that are checked the greater the quantity of inferior pride. Take a moment to repent to God for the different types of pride you have identified and ask Him to change this excessive self-focus.

STEP C: ANGER

1. What is the pattern of your anger? What things do you typically get angry about?

Circle any of the above anger-triggers that are based on a selfish motive.

2. What injustice have you experienced?

3. Who has committed this injustice toward you? Write down their names. Ask the Holy Spirit to reveal any other people or groups of people you are angry with and write their names down also.

If this anger remains too long without being resolved our feelings will tend to change over time, as you can see by this timeline of the typical process of anger:

Initial feelings → anger (or wrath) → bitterness/contempt → hate → cynicism/indifference

Ultimately, cynicism and indifference are forms of repressed anger. What or who we are cynical about will probably be the circumstances or people we were once angry with, and the anger has cooled into indifference or cynicism. For instance, if somebody from a certain country or racial group hurt you, you might develop a critical spirit toward anyone from that country or act indifferently toward anyone from that particular race if you have failed to deal well with the initial hurt.

Take a moment and ask the Holy Spirit to reveal to you which people you are cynical toward or are indifferent to. Write down their names or the group of people they represent.

Now ask the Holy Spirit to reveal where your anger first started with each of these names or groups of people.

Did anybody model unhealthy anger to you as you were growing up? It may be helpful to ask the Holy Spirit what the origin of unhealthy anger in your life is. I did this with a friend of mine, and he sensed it was the year 1981. I asked if this was when he was quite young, and he surprised me by saying it was before he was born! I was about to dismiss it when I felt the Holy Spirit prompt me to press further. My friend asked the Holy Spirit what this meant, and he saw a picture of his father and grandfather playing a card game and watched as his grandfather acted spitefully to his father. My friend realized that this had been a pattern in their home growing up; his father had also acted spitefully toward him, and it made him angry. He forgave both his grandfather and father for their part in him developing unhealthy anger patterns, and it brought great inner healing to my friend.

For all the names you have written down above, use the process from chapter 5 to forgive all of them from your heart.

Anger toward God

One of the things I do in addition to being a pastor is business coaching. I was once with a client in his offices, and we were working through a relationship that had cooled. As my client realized that his indifference toward the once-close friendship stemmed from an unresolved issue, he realized he was actually quite angry with his friend. My client was a Christian so I took him through the forgiveness process in this book and, as he dealt with his hurt, he realized that this relationship was an exact mirror of his current relationship with God. He knew he ought to spend time with God (through Bible reading, prayer, etc.), but he didn't want to. It dawned on him that he might be angry with God. However, he quickly rationalized that he couldn't be angry with God who had done so much for him, could he?

A lot of Christians feel guilty about feelings of anger toward God, but maybe the guilt is pointing to something beneath the anger. The psalmists show us a healthy way to deal with feelings of anger towards God. In any relationship, healing comes when we talk through hurts and admit how we feel. If you feel you may have anger toward God, or if you definitely know that you do, there are many things you can do, such as repress it, deny it, or speak to other people about it. But instead, can I suggest that you do as the psalmists have shown us, and tell God about your anger directly? He knows it already, but by speaking to Him about it you are choosing to engage with Him relationally.

When the psalmists cry out to God about their anger, they are nonetheless respectful toward God, acknowledging that they are the created talking to their Creator. A healthy pattern I have noticed in several psalms is that they conclude in worship, even after they have expressed their anger.

Read the six verses of Psalm 13 and then follow its pattern to express your anger to God. (If you are a creative type you may want to write your own psalm to God, patterned on Psalm 13.)

> *How long, O Lord? Will you forget me forever? How long will you hide your face from me? How long must I take counsel in my soul and have sorrow in my heart all the day? How long shall my enemy be exalted over me? Consider and answer me, O Lord my God; light up my eyes, lest I sleep the sleep of death, lest my enemy say, "I have prevailed over him," lest my foes rejoice because I am shaken. But I have trusted in your steadfast love; my heart shall rejoice in your salvation. I will sing to the Lord, because he has dealt bountifully with me.*
>
> (Psalm 13:1–6)

Once you have expressed your anger to God, you may feel that there are things you can say sorry for that were previously hidden from you. Take a moment and do so. If you find it difficult to worship Him, ask God to remind you of His goodness toward you and then respond with thanks for the things He shows you.

Anger toward self

As well as being angry with God or others I find that many people are angry with themselves. For instance, if you asked people if they liked their bodies, many would respond with a definite negative. Some would be more forceful and say that they hate their bodies. Hatred is one of the emotions that follows all anger, and when I have probed people about this, the anger is commonly expressed toward God for making their bodies a certain way, or their anger is toward themselves for not taking better care of their bodies. Either way, to be healthy, this anger needs to be processed. If you sense that your anger is toward God then I suggest that you go back to the section above. If you have anger toward yourself, then the best way to deal with this well is to turn it into repentance before God. For example, "God, I am sorry that I haven't looked after my body as I should. Specifically, I ask forgiveness for _____. Please forgive me and teach me how to both live differently and see my body differently."

Reflect on these questions: Do you have any other forms of anger toward yourself? What is root cause of this anger? Follow the same pattern as above.

KEY POINTS

1. Allowing our love to become disordered can have negative effects on our health.

2. Two symptoms of disordered love that are particularly dangerous to our health are pride (excessive self-love) and unrighteous anger (getting angry for selfish reasons).

3. Identifying and recognizing these symptoms in ourselves allows us to ask God to change us—which may lead to significant health improvements.

CHAPTER 8:

UNCOVERING HIDDEN SYMPTOMS

"There are things which a man is afraid to tell even to himself, and every decent man has a number of such things stored away in his mind."
—*Fyodor Dostoevsky*
Nineteenth-century Russian novelist

Ellen was the second of four children. When she was six months old, her father was diagnosed with schizophrenia, a severe mental illness characterized by delusions, hallucinations, and hearing voices. During her early years, he was in and out of mental hospitals. Her first memory of visiting him in a hospital is from when she was five years old. She wore a new dress and brought him a gift, but he hardly recognized who she was, and threw the gift away. Half-way through their time together, he got up and walked away, without explanation. She felt terribly rejected and a fear gripped her. What if people found out how strange her father was? Over the years, this fear took on different forms, including nightmares and being terrified of the dark.

Her father's doctors told the family that schizophrenia had a genetic component and that it was likely one the four children would suffer from mental illness at some point. Her family described Ellen as a sensitive child, and she felt they had decided that if anyone were going to develop a mental illness, it would be her.

Ellen never spoke about her fears, and this created an inner torment that no amount of counselling could solve. When she reached fourteen years of age, she was hospitalized for the first time. She had been having difficulty sleeping, and she was admitted for a week of what was called sleep therapy. Through medications she was kept asleep day and night and only woken up temporarily at meal times. This seemed to alleviate her symptoms and give her some respite, but the following year, it happened again. On this occasion she was diagnosed with clinical depression. She was given medications that had severe side effects—swinging her between feeling like a zombie and feeling intense anxiety. This became a pattern in Ellen's life; every March she would start to be hyperactive, fail to sleep, be admitted for sleep therapy, and then improve.

When she was sixteen she described her fear as a monster, and she thought to herself that she would rather be dead than live with it. When she reached the age of eighteen, her difficulty sleeping became such a problem, she resorted to stealing away from class in order to find somewhere quiet to sleep during the day. She had also started to hear sporadic voices in her head that told her to do strange things, such as singing loudly during a quiet part of a church service. At times she also got the idea that she wasn't a high school student but actually a health specialist. Because of this she only wore white and thought she had a stethoscope around her neck. On other occasions she thought she could read people's minds.

Things came to a head when one weekend she couldn't sleep at all. She lay at home in a catatonic-like state, too tired to move, but unable to sleep. Her mother drove her to the nearest mental hospital. Ellen felt helpless as she watched the psychiatrist talk about her to her mother. She feared being institutionalized like her dad, but it now looked as though what she feared most was about to happen. The psychiatrist said that although Ellen didn't have all the typical symptoms of schizophrenia, she had enough to make the diagnosis. Speaking as though she wasn't in the room, he told Ellen's mom that Ellen would probably be a "vegetable" by twenty-two years old, would not marry or have children, and would likely remain in the hospital for the rest of her life.

Her mother had packed a suitcase for Ellen before they had travelled to the hospital, which Ellen took as a sign that her mother had lost faith in her recovery. Against her wishes, Ellen was admitted. No one visited her, and her parents wouldn't chat on the phone for long. Ellen, who had become a Christian at a youth group when she was sixteen, cried out to God, asking, "Is this why I was born?" to which she didn't seem to get a reply.

Later on, she remembers sitting on a bench and asking God to please, please, speak to her. This time, peace came over her mind, and she felt God say that though her enemies are many, she did not have to be afraid anymore because He would rescue her. He would be a shield around her and would lift up her head. She later discovered this was found in the beginning of the third psalm.

Hugely grateful that God had finally spoken, she took Him at His word and declared that He was in charge from that point on. A calm came over her, so noticeable that one of her doctors experimentally took her off all of her medications. A few weeks later, a panel was convened, and they told her that although they couldn't explain her dramatic change, they had decided she was fit to be discharged.

Once she left the hospital, she continued to live normally. Two years later, she met her husband to whom she finally voiced her various deep-seated fears for the very first time. Ellen remembers something dramatic happening as she voiced them—as though their hold on her simply broke. From that time on, Ellen learned to live differently. She went on to have three children, and in spite of having missed out on her final year of high school, recently completed a degree in psychology. She and her husband are active leaders in their church, and Ellen often shares her testimony, speaking of God's power to set people free from fear and its devastating effects.

FEAR AND HEALTH

The presence of fear in our lives can have big domino effect on our health. Perhaps we fear the side effects of a certain drug, so we don't take it, or we fear what a health professional may tell us, so we delay making an appointment. If our symptom is a sore throat, then the consequences probably won't be significant. But if we're too afraid to visit a doctor and our symptoms are caused by a heart attack, then the consequences are a matter of life and death!

A team of nurses investigated just that question—why certain patients delayed going to the hospital when they had cardiac symptoms.[143] They discovered a number of fears amongst their reasons. People delayed getting help because they were fearful of losing a healthy identity. They also delayed because they were fearful of the effect that a heart attack would have on friends and family. In some, their delay was less rationalized, saying that a general panic prevented them from calling for help earlier.

These delays can be costly. Currently, 30 percent of people who have a heart attack die from it, but half of those deaths occurred before the patient reached the hospital.[144] Studies have shown that early intervention (such as taking aspirin at home or getting to the

143. C. Nymark, et al., "Emotions delay care-seeking in patients with an acute myocardial infarction," National Center for Biotechnology Information, http://www.ncbi.nlm.nih.gov/pubmed/23341477 (accessed 29 May 2015).
144. A. Maziar Zafari, MD, PhD, et al., "Myocardial Infarction," Medscape, http://emedicine.medscape.com/article/155919-overview#aw2aab6b2b7aa (accessed 22 April 2015).

hospital sooner) can dramatically change the outcome. Quite literally, when the symptoms start, the clock is ticking, and every minute counts. Any delay, caused by fear or anything else, can have consequences that are irreversible and immensely regrettable.

It is not just in-the-moment fear that can damage our health; we can also experience poor health through longstanding fears. For instance, fear is one of the reasons why we live in stress; all of the negative health effects from stress that we saw in chapter 3 can be rooted in longstanding fear. Fear is also the main drive behind obsessive compulsive disorder (OCD), in which victims are often so fearful of germs that they scrub themselves frequently or are so fearful of feeling out of control that they obsess about their external environment. Fear of being sick can also result in hypochondria, where we over-investigate the most minor of symptoms. The stress that comes from this fear of sickness often leads to its own sickness.

In 2005, Johan Denollet, a professor of medical psychology at Tilburg University in the Netherlands, coined the phrase "Type D personality" ("D" stood for "distress"). People with Type D personality are characterized by worry, gloominess, and social isolation. He said that the social isolation is often caused by a fear of rejection by others, so it is fair to say that people with this personality are characterized by fear, and it should probably be called the "fear" personality type. Studies have shown that the presence of Type D personality is very bad for your health; people with this personality have four times the risk of having a heart attack than those without it.[145] Worse still, if people do have a heart attack, those with Type D also take longer to recover than other patients.[146] It is safe to say this fear-associated personality is not a helpful one to have when it comes to heart disease.

---

145. J. Denollet et al., "Personality as independent predictor of long-term mortality in patients with coronary heart disease," *Lancet* 347, no. 8999 (February, 1996): 417–421.

146. J. Denollet, J. Vaes, and D. L. Brutsaert, "Inadequate response to treatment in coronary heart disease: adverse effects of type D personality and younger age on 5-year prognosis and quality of life" *Circulation* 102, no. 6 (August 2000): 630–635.

Fear can also stop people from receiving supernatural healing. Jesus specifically stated that anxiety hinders faith[147] and, as we'll see in chapter 10, faith is an important part of seeking God for supernatural healing. Not dealing with anxious thoughts can have significant health effects. I once received healing for back pain, but I almost refused to receive prayer for fear of what other people would think.

Fear eats away at faith, and it gets in the way of us connecting with God.

Disconnection from God is probably the biggest reason for fear's bad health effects. At its root, fear is a denial that God is close to us and able to help us. Consider some of the common fears. Fear of failure is actually an acknowledgment deep down that God won't, or can't, help us find success.[148] Fear of loneliness is actually an acknowledgment that we don't believe God can either be a Friend to us or provide a healthy community for us.[149] Fear of death actually means that we don't believe that God will be with us when we die or that He doesn't have something better waiting for the believer after our body passes away.

Dr. Andrew Selle, a Christian counselor and minister, says that fear actually reveals our deepest longings. He says this:

> Fear is the reverse of desire. You are afraid of dying: you want to live. You fear your children will fail in school: you want them to succeed. You are afraid of looking foolish: you want others to see you as wise and spiritually mature. You fear rejection: you want acceptance.[150]

It is not wrong to have desires, but when our desires lead us to crippling fear, something is not right within us. The Bible says

---

147. See Matthew 6:28–30.
148. Which is in contrast to what He promises us in Proverbs 3:3–4.
149. See John 15:15; Psalm 68:6.
150. A. H. Selle, "The Bridge over Troubled Waters: Overcoming Crippling Fear by Faith and Love," *Journal of Biblical Counseling* (Fall 2002): 36.

that we are to fear God[151] and, taking Selle's definition, that means ultimately we are to desire God. As we have discussed previously, when our desire for created things becomes greater than our desire for our Creator, things go wrong. In this case we open ourselves up to unhealthy fear, which Paul commands us to be ruthless in dealing with.[152] Unresolved, unhealthy fear leads to two things: comfort, because we look for something to help us escape when fear overtakes us, and control, because we look for ways to take control of our out-of-control situation.

The Oscar-winning actor Robin Williams was loved by millions around the world for comedic roles in such films as *Good Morning Vietnam*, *Patch Adams*, and *Mrs. Doubtfire*. He was also very moving in more serious roles such as the psychologist in *Good Will Hunting* and the schoolteacher in *Dead Poets Society*. However, success didn't necessarily bring happiness for Williams, who had an on-again, off-again decades-long battle with addictions. During the 1970s and '80s he admitted to an addiction to cocaine, and in both 2006 and 2014 he was admitted to rehabilitation centers for alcoholism. After a period of sobriety, in an interview in *The Guardian* newspaper (UK), he was asked if the trigger for turning back to alcohol was the death of his close friend and former Superman actor, Christopher Reeve. He replied: "No…it's more selfish than that. It's just literally being afraid. And you think, oh, this will ease the fear. And it doesn't." The interviewer asked what he was afraid of and Williams replied: "Everything. It's just a general all-round arggghhh. It's fearfulness and anxiety."[153]

Sometime in his early sixties, Williams was diagnosed with the early stages of Parkinson's disease, a degenerative disease of the nervous system that is characterized by depression initially, followed by progressive dementia. Sadly, there is no cure for this

---

151. See 2 Corinthians 5:11.
152. See Philippians 4:6–7.
153. Quoted in Decca Aitkenhead, "Robin Williams," *The Guardian*, September 20, 2010, http://www.theguardian.com/film/2010/sep/20/robin-williams-worlds-greatest-dad-alcohol-drugs (accessed 22 April 2015).

disease, and the medications available only delay the progression of symptoms. As the disease progresses, the person gradually loses control of his or her reasoning and memory. On top of his struggle with addictions, it seems likely this future was too much to bear for Williams; on August 11, 2014, aged sixty-three, he definitively took control of his situation and hung himself.

The health effects of addictive substances, legal or otherwise, are numerous (mental health disease, cancers, etc.), but the feeling of helplessness that longstanding fear can generate has even larger effects on us spiritually. If we fail to know in our heart that God is in control of our situation, we may try to take control of our own situation in our own strength, or worse, try to take control by controlling others.

Attempting to control people or circumstances in response to fear is a behavioral pattern that can run through families; modeled by the parents or older siblings, it's learned by the younger ones and eventually passed on. Similar to abusive situations, where often the abused becomes the abuser, often the controlled person often becomes the controller, subtly using emotions and circumstance to manipulate a desired behavior in others. This is a big problem spiritually; the effects of this kind of control-taking can be felt in the office, in relationships, in friendships, in careers, or even with strangers. It is something we need to deal with because it prevents us from connecting to God in those moments.

THE OCCULT

A desire for control is one the reasons that draws people into trying out the occult. The word "occult" is derived from the Latin word *occultus*, meaning "secret" or "hidden," and I use it broadly to refer to any practices that seek to connect to the spiritual realm outside of what God has permitted. Connection to the spiritual realm not mediated through one of the members of the Trinity opens us up to demonic oppression, which may manifest as sickness.

Grace's Story

Grace came to my wife and me for counseling. She had just got engaged and recently discovered that her future mother-in-law was into spiritual practices that didn't sit well with her. Grace told us that she had been waking up screaming after bad dreams and this coincided with occasions when her future mother-in-law had told her she had sent "angels" to help her. We prayed for the oppression to stop but we also told Grace that she needed to speak with her fiancé's mother and explain why these practices were not helpful. Fortunately Grace's fiancé stepped in and spoke to his mother and asked her to stop sending the spirits, and the night terrors stopped.

In Luke's gospel we read of a woman who was healed from a crippling postural disease that was specifically caused by an evil spirit.[154] In a similar vein, Matthew tells us of a mute man that was healed by Jesus after he had received his condition through demonic oppression.[155] In what appears to be a judgment on Elymas' sorcery, God made him blind after he tried to oppose Paul's preaching of the gospel.[156]

Out of desperation, or through seeing others getting healed, some long-term sick people dangerously experiment with occultic healing methods. For instance, the healing technique Reiki is based on an ancient Buddhist method of laying hands to channel healing energy to an area of the body that is ill. Receiving any supernatural healing outside of the authority of Jesus will always have a demonic power source, and Reiki, just to name one, is a cause of much spiritual oppression. A person using Reiki may initially feel some relief from the symptoms, and the condition may

---

154. See Luke 13:10–13.
155. See Matthew 9:32–33.
156. See Acts 13:8–12.

even seem to resolve, but they will always be left in a much worse place spiritually.

Sophia's Story

Sophia was sitting in our lounge as part of our church's young adults group when I noticed that she put her hand up to shade her eyes from the light. I paused the discussion and asked if something was wrong, and she explained she had developed a migraine and was feeling nauseous. Nina, a girl in the group, remarked that she had also suddenly felt nauseous but that this had gone away as soon as Sophia started speaking. Nina got the sense that God was highlighting something about Sophia's nausea. Sophia was new to our group, and she turned out to be quite a troubled girl. She explained that the nausea had first happened on one occasion when she had got angry with God and, out of feelings of despair, had decided to convert to another religion. She went through an unusual ceremony where a lady chanted over her in Arabic and then anointed her with oil. As the lady placed the oil on Sophia, she vomited. Her migraines and nausea had been present, on and off, ever since that ceremony. I explained to Sophia that there seemed to be a connection between the process she had gone through and her current feelings. I led her through a prayer of repentance for turning her back on Jesus and for choosing to go through the particular conversion process, and we asked Jesus to break off any of the effects of this. Instantly the nausea and the migraine lifted, and she said she felt both lighter and far more peaceful.

It is impossible to list all of the occultic healing practices that are available, but in general anything that has a New Age or traditional Eastern spiritual basis will ultimately derive any supernatural power demonically. Examples of this include new age healing crystals, shamanistic healing, psychic healing, aura adjustment, yoga, reflexology, etc. In Africa, this includes any healing processes carried out by witch doctors.

Worryingly, some of these unhealthy spiritual practices are becoming accepted in conventional medicine. Whenever something new or unfamiliar is offered, it is always important to research the underlying source of healing. For example, traditional Chinese acupuncture is based on energy redirection derived from a Buddhist philosophy of the body. Chinese herbal medicine is a whole system of medicine that is becoming popular, but it operates on a similar Buddhist spiritual foundation to traditional Chinese acupuncture. The Buddhist component makes it problematic for Christians, and participation in it may be spiritually harmful.

While participation in occultic healing practices is one cause of demonic oppression, any participation in the occult will affect us spiritually. At the end of the chapter, I will outline a process on how to ask God to free you from this if you have ever participated in anything occultic, but let me first show you how the occult can hold such power.

THE SIGNIFICANCE OF COVENANTS

God has formed a number of covenants with us. A covenant is a binding agreement between two parties. For instance, in Genesis chapter 6, God told Noah, *"I will establish my covenant with you"* (Genesis 6:18). This agreement specified that Noah was to bring into the ark a proportion of animals and food from the earth, and, in return, God would keep him and his family safe from the floodwaters that God was about to send. As Noah found out, keeping covenant with God resulted in life and blessings.

Conversely, as Adam had already discovered, breaking a covenant with God is a serious matter and results in curses. In Genesis chapters 1 and 2, we see that God made a covenant with Adam that included all of his descendants. The covenant outlined that if we would obey God, in exchange God would give us dominion over the earth and a death-free existence.[157] Adam broke that covenant and, as his descendants, we are still living with the effect of the curses that resulted.[158] In a similar way, through Moses, God established a detailed covenant with the Israelites. This covenant listed very specific expectations of obedience.[159] Maintaining the covenant would result in many blessings, but breaking the covenant would lead to very specific curses.[160]

When people look to access supernatural healing outside of God, whether they know it or not, they effectively enter into a covenant in the spiritual realm. In exchange for demonically sourced healing, they give demons certain access. While the magnitude of the covenant is vastly smaller than the covenants God has made with us, the covenants still carry spiritual significance and need to be repented of in order to receive freedom. Thankfully, Jesus defeated evil through the cross, and if we have entered into covenant with Him (through His vastly superior new covenant), then He can grant us forgiveness and freedom from all and any covenants we may have made with darkness. His covenant trumps all other covenants. Additionally, because He became a curse on our behalf,[161] He has the power to nullify any associated curses.

Daniel's Story

Daniel's dad had been a Freemason. One day, as his mother was receiving prayer, Daniel sat in his school class and, as usual, saw the words in front of him jumbled up. Daniel had dyslexia and only read with great difficultly. However, in that moment something incredible happened. The words sorted themselves out before his eyes, and he could suddenly read normally. A few miles away his mother had just asked God to break off any spiritual effects on her

---

157. See Genesis 1:28–31; 2:16–17
158. See Genesis 3:16–19.
159. See Exodus 20:1–17 and the whole book of Leviticus.
160. See Deuteronomy 11:26–32; 28.
161. See Galatians 3:13.

or her family that occurred from her husband's former involvement in freemasonry. The result of this prayer was that Daniel was dramatically cured of dyslexia.

Secret societies, such as freemasonry, can be particularly problematic because participants form a number of spiritual covenants. For instance, to become a Master Mason, an oath is taken to maintain the secrets of freemasonry to the point of death. Breaking this oath incurs many curses. Freemasonry oaths specifically claim to take precedence over other covenants, including marriage (symbolically the wedding ring is removed prior to swearing the oath), and, importantly for Christians, Jesus' new covenant.

Freemasonry, and its related societies, consistently claims not to be a religion. However, the presence of a temple, religious services, rituals, and a process for eternal salvation (through good works) all seem to have the markings of a religion. Through assisting people to renounce the oaths of freemasonry, I have seen people gain a lot of spiritual freedom, even when they themselves haven't participated in freemasonry, but some family authority figure has.

A former colleague of mine had severe depression and her psychiatrist, after already placing her on a combination of three medications, said the next step was electro-convulsive therapy (ECT). Not liking the prospect of having electrodes placed on her brain and a high voltage of electricity sent through them, she asked for Christian counseling. This was moderately helpful, but the real breakthrough came when she went to visit her parents and learned that a close family member had been very involved in freemasonry. A minister came to the house and prayed for the family to be free of any unhelpful influence this had caused, and her depression dramatically lifted. Very quickly she came off her medication and remains free of medication to this day—never needing ECT.

SEXUAL SIN

The apostle Paul tells us that sexual sin is different to other sins because it is not just a sin against God but also a sin against our own bodies:

> *Flee from sexual immorality. Every other sin a person commits is outside the body, but the sexually immoral person sins against his own body. Or do you not know that your body is a temple of the Holy Spirit within you, whom you have from God? You are not your own, for you were bought with a price. So glorify God in your body.*   (1 Corinthians 6:18–20)

When we have sex, the Bible tells us, our souls connect, and God designed these soul connections, more commonly called soul ties, to be a good thing.[162] We see from Adam and Eve that sex was created to join people together,[163] and God's plan was that sex would be carried out in the context of a life-long marriage covenant. The marriage covenant creates a place where emotional nakedness and physical nakedness can occur concurrently. To help bond the marriage, God created sex as a covenant glue.[164] Every time a couple has sex, their souls are increasingly knit together.

Grant's Story

Grant was in a small, topical Bible study for some of the young men in our church. One evening, as we looked at Ephesians 6 and discussed spiritual warfare, Grant started looking ill, and I noticed his breathing getting heavier. It was as though some external force was pushing him down. Our group stopped the Bible study and asked Grant if he felt all right. He wasn't—he was quite distressed and started panicking, not understanding what was happening. Grant had become a Christian a few years earlier but ever since had suffered from vivid nightmares

---

162. See Genesis 34:2–3.
163. See Genesis 2:24.
164. See Ephesians 5:31.

that woke him up in a cold sweat. Sometimes he would scream, loud enough to wake up his dad in another room. Grant had learned to live with the situation but was now experiencing something new—the same terror that visited him during the night was now afflicting him in broad daylight, surrounded by friends, in a Bible study.

We commanded any evil to stop, and our group asked God to reveal why Grant was experiencing this. I felt God show me that there was a sexual link, and I asked Grant if he had ever broken soul ties with people he had slept with before becoming a Christian. He answered he hadn't, so I led him through the prayer to break soul ties (located at the end of this chapter). During the prayer time, when he came to one particular ex-girlfriend, he found he couldn't say the prayer. He said it felt like something was holding his tongue. Our group sang a worship song, the grip seemed to loosen, and Grant just managed to say the prayer. Instantly the pressure lifted, and Grant started to feel much better. Grant told us that this particular ex-girlfriend had been involved in the occult, and Grant realized that through having a sexual relationship with this girl, it had opened him up to demonic oppression.

When I was a pastor in a young adults' church, I remember receiving an email from a visiting couple asking for counsel. They had recently had a nasty falling out with each other and had broken up, but neither of them seemed able to move on. As I read through their story, I knew what must have happened. Sure enough, in the second paragraph of the email they explained they used to live together and had been intimate regularly. Sex joins. It has a way of connecting us at a number of levels. If you have committed to be together for the rest of your life, this is a good thing. But if you haven't, it can be quite problematic. This couple was torn; because of their large fight, they didn't feel they could commit to each other, but emotionally they couldn't move on.

The book of Genesis recounts a time when Shechem the Hivite forced himself on Jacob's daughter Dinah, and, tragically, raped her.[165] After the event, the Bible tells us *"his soul was drawn"* to her. Though he demonstrated a total disregard of Dinah's feelings and rights, a connection had been made, and he asked his father to make arrangements for them to marry. While Shechem thought he was in love with Dinah before he raped her, after they had sex he decided that he couldn't be without her. In a similar way Paul warns the Corinthian church that having sex with a prostitute creates an unhealthy joining.[166] Not only do we sin against God, but by not following God's sexual ethic, we bring much unnecessary complication to our earthly relationships.

While soul ties can be formed sexually, they can also form emotionally. For example, the Bible says that David and Jonathan's close friendship resulted in the soul of Jonathan being *"knit to the soul of David"* (1 Samuel 18:1). However, not all emotional soul ties are healthy, and if identified, need to be broken. Take, for instance, the unhealthy emotional connection that can occur between some bosses and their assistants or secretaries, who are willing to work at all hours of the day and night at the request of their boss, but then come to the realization that they have been taken advantage of when they change jobs. If you feel you may have formed an unhealthy soul tie (whether sexually or emotionally) with someone, there is process to break them at the end of the chapter.

It is not just the formation of unhealthy soul ties that can result from ignoring God's sexual ethic. As a medical student, I have been to enough sexual health clinics to see the many and varied terrible health consequences that unwise sexual choices produce. Sexually transmitted infections abound, and while many of them can be treated with antibiotics, others cannot. In fact, because some are treatable, it can lure people into a false sense of security despite the fact that many other sexually transmitted infections

---

165. See Genesis 34:1–4.
166. See 1 Corinthians 6:16.

are incurable and plague the patient for the rest of their life. For instance, while chlamydia, syphilis, gonorrhea, and trichomoniasis can all be resolved with a short course of antibiotics, genital herpes, genital warts, and hepatitis B do not currently have an effective treatment. Even chlamydia can be problematic, because infection doesn't always result in symptoms, and, in women, if the infection is left untreated, it may cause Pelvic Inflammatory Disease (an infection involving the reproductive organs), which is one of the most common causes of infertility in the Western world.

South Africa, the country where I live, has more than five million people currently infected with Human Immunodeficiency Virus (HIV). That is 17 percent of the adult population, or just over one in five adults that I meet. In the Southern African region, the number of people who are HIV positive is at least twice as high as in other parts of the world, and sometimes more like five times as high.[167] Unlike in Europe and the United States, where HIV is most commonly transmitted through high-risk behavior (injecting drug use, anal intercourse, etc.), in Southern Africa, HIV is most commonly passed on through heterosexual sex.

While South Africans and their neighbors do not have more sexual partners than people in other parts of the world, the reason HIV has spread so rapidly is due to the all-too-common practice here of multiple, concurrent sexual partnerships. In other words, unlike the majority of the rest of the world, many Southern Africans have more than one sexual partner at a time, sometimes even three or four fairly longstanding partnerships. This practice creates a mass of interconnected sexual networks, which have been well-documented, and these create fertile ground for the rapid spread of HIV.

Cervical cancer is another disease that is often the result of unhealthy sexual practice.[168] This cancer is generated after infec-

---

167. See http://en.wikipedia.org/?title=List_of_countries_by_HIV/AIDS_adult_prevalence_rate.
168. A study in 1952 looked at 13,000 sexually non-active nuns and not one of them had symptoms of the disease.

tion with the human papilloma virus, a sexually transmitted virus. Infection by the virus leads to changes in the DNA of the cells of a women's cervix (the neck of the womb). With enough DNA changes, a cell becomes cancerous and multiplies uncontrollably.

Sadly, all these conditions would effectively disappear in a generation or two if everybody in the world followed God's sexual ethic and kept sex within the confines of a marriage covenant. Our failure to do so has led to a heavy burden of sexually transmitted disease around the world. It has also led to millions of lives being terminated prematurely.

ABORTION

I write this next section with heaviness in my heart, knowing that the emotion associated with this topic cannot be properly related to with the words available. However, as a pastor, and knowing the spiritual problems that this issue can create for people who are seeking God for healing, this is an important blockage to healing that needs to be addressed.

In Leviticus, God commands the Israelites not to sacrifice their children to Molech.[169] So serious was this decree that God issued a penalty of excommunication followed by death for anyone who disobeyed it.[170] Molech was an Ammonite god who received worship through people bringing their children and sacrificing them to him on his altar;[171] a practice so terrible that God told the prophet Jeremiah that *"nor did it enter in to my mind, that they should do this abomination"* (Jeremiah 32:35). The Psalms tells us this practice, like any idolatry, was actually worship of demons.[172] When the king of Moab was losing a battle against the Israelites,

---

169. See Leviticus 18:21.
170. See Leviticus 20:2.
171. See 1 Kings 11:7; 2 Kings 23:10.
172. See Psalm 106:36–37.

he sacrificed his own son in order to successfully recruit demonic help and save the battle.[173]

When I was a recently qualified hospital doctor, I had to face the fact that a mistake I made contributed to the death of one of my patients. As one of the junior doctors on the team, it was my responsibility to take regular blood samples of a patient who was on warfarin, a medication used to reduce the blood's clotting ability. Because of urgent situations, this routine job was placed further down on my priority list and was completed later than it should have been. A senior colleague assumed I had checked the blood already and prescribed the patient's usual dose. We were only to find out too late that the level was too high. For the next week or so we tried to bring down the blood levels, but the patient was quite sick. His liver and kidneys were not functioning as they should have been and couldn't reduce the warfarin levels. One afternoon my buzzer went off to signify that I needed to rush to a patient in a dangerous condition. As I raced to the location I discovered my patient had started bleeding uncontrollably. Because of the high levels of warfarin, his blood wasn't clotting, and despite being taken to emergency room, he died.

I told myself that he was very sick and that he wouldn't have lived much longer anyway, but I couldn't shake the fact that my actions had contributed to his death. In our training, one of our tutors had soberly said that the inevitable effect of human error within a pressurized work environment would lead to us all contributing to someone's death at some point in our careers, and I tried to console myself with this statement, but the guilt still remained. It was only when a senior colleague, seeing that I was burdened by the situation, told me, "You need to accept that you and your colleague made a mistake and this resulted in a person's death," that I could come to terms with the situation. My actions had killed another human being. Accepting this enabled me to fully repent before God and correctly work through the situation.

173. See 2 Kings 3:26–27.

Sadly, in many societies today, you do not have to be a health care professional to cause the medical termination of life. While we may not place newborn babies on pagan altars, our legal systems have made it acceptable, and technology has made it possible, to bring about similar outcomes with our unborn children through the process of abortion. Passionate arguments are made that women should be able to do what they want with their bodies. Anger-inducing cases of horrific rape are used to try and justify the killing of intra-uterine fetuses, but all around the world the result is the same: millions of innocent lives are terminated before they can even see the light of day by a medicalized form of killing.

In the United States, approximately one million abortions occur legally each year.[174] Only 1 percent of these are prompted in response to rape, with the vast majority being carried out for reasons of lifestyle and convenience. The doctors that carry them out, the partners and family members that push for them, and the mothers who allow them, can only push aside the guilt from participating in the killing of an innocent human being if they convince themselves that they are not actually killing an innocent human being. No one can deny the fetus isn't innocent, so the only option available is to deny that the fetus is human. However, God told the prophet Jeremiah, *"Before I formed you in the womb I knew you...I appointed you a prophet to the nations"* (Jeremiah 1:5). The psalmist tell us that God knits us together in the womb and that God writes all our days in His book.[175] God, at least, seems to know a lot about our humanity while we are still a fetus. If we are Christians, we must not look to society to tell us what is acceptable, but instead we must look to God.

Like my situation with my former patient, it is only if we admit the full horror of the situation that we will be able to deal with any

---

174. Guttmacher Institute, "Fact Sheet: Induced Abortion in the United States," July 2014, http://www.guttmacher.org/pubs/fb_induced_abortion.html (accessed 29 May 2015).

175. See Psalm 139:13, 16.

guilt that we have. Western society tells us abortion just removes unwanted parts of our bodies, similar to any other operation, but God sees it quite differently, telling the Israelites who participated in Molech worship: *"you slaughtered my children and delivered them up as an offering by fire"* (Ezekiel 16:21).

We may see the children that we bear as belonging to us, but God sees it differently. They belong to Him. If we choose to shorten their lives, then we ultimately sin against God and need to repent. If you have participated in abortion you may try, as I did with my patient, to justify what happened or to minimize your part in the process, but our consciences hold us accountable and we can only be freed when we acknowledge the horror of an innocent human dying, and bring that horror with repentance to God.

Some people struggle with depression and even suicidal thoughts in response to an abortion. I have also found that abortion can sometimes harm people's ability to conceive—until it has been repented of.

While the act of abortion has huge spiritual consequence, the good news is that God's grace is bigger and He is able and willing to forgive our actions—even when they resulted in the death of others. If this chapter has brought up some unpleasant feelings or memories, you may want to pause for a moment and ask God to strengthen you and minister to you before you continue.

PRACTICAL STEPS

STEP A: SETTING THE SCENE

+ Choose a place where you won't be disturbed.

+ Choose a moment when you will not be interrupted.

+ Turn off your cell phone.

+ If you feel it would be helpful, ask a trusted Christian friend to be with you and quietly pray as you go through the process.

STEP B: FEAR

+ What fears do you commonly experience?
    - ❑ Fear of failure
    - ❑ Fear of disapproval
    - ❑ Fear of illness
    - ❑ Fear of heights
    - ❑ Fear of dying
    - ❑ Fear of being alone
    - ❑ Fear of poverty
    - ❑ Fear of the dark
    - ❑ Fear of rejection
    - ❑ Fear of secrets being exposed
    - ❑ Fear of spiders or snakes
    - ❑ Fear of dogs or other animals
    - ❑ Other _____

For all the fears you have checked, write down the desire that is the reversal of the fear. (For example, if you have a fear of failure, it may indicate the presence of a desire to succeed; if you have a fear of heights, it may indicate the presence of a desire to feel safe/in control.)

Take each of the desires you have listed, and ask the Holy Spirit to reveal whether these are too important in your life. If so, take a moment to say sorry to God and ask Him to help you put the desires in their correct place.

STEP C: THE OCCULT

Check if you have been involved, actively or passively, with any of the following:

Occult healing:

- ❏ Reiki
- ❏ Healing Crystals
- ❏ Shamanistic healing
- ❏ Witch doctor
- ❏ Psychic healing
- ❏ Aura adjustment
- ❏ Yoga
- ❏ Polarity therapy
- ❏ Shiatsu
- ❏ Qigong
- ❏ Biofeedback

Other occult practices:

- ❏ Tarot cards
- ❏ Ouija board
- ❏ Séances / automatic writing
- ❏ Astrology/horoscopes
- ❏ Casting spells/curses
- ❏ Clairvoyance
- ❏ Spirit guides
- ❏ Fortune-telling
- ❏ Palm reading
- ❏ Ancestral worship
- ❏ Other: _____

184 I'm Sick, Now What?

Depending on the depth of involvement, the following occult practices will probably need somebody experienced in seeing people set free to pray with you:

- ❏ Black or white magic
- ❏ Paganism
- ❏ Satanism
- ❏ Astral-projection
- ❏ Telepathy
- ❏ Witchcraft/Wiccan

For each one, pray: "God, I repent of my involvement in _____ and ask that You remove any bad spiritual effect that has resulted from my involvement."

STEP D: FREEMASONRY

Have a look at the following secret societies associated with freemasonry. If you or anybody in your immediate family have been involved in these, or other societies where covenants are entered into, I suggest you use the prayer listed underneath.

Societies connected to Freemasonry:

- ❏ Holy Royal Arch
- ❏ The Shrine
- ❏ Royal Order of Jesters
- ❏ Tall Cedars of Lebanon
- ❏ The Grotto
- ❏ Knights Templar
- ❏ Royal Arch Masonry
- ❏ Societas Rosicurciana
- ❏ Association of Youth Hope of the Fraternity
- ❏ Cryptic Masonry

- ❑ Order of St. Thomas of Acon
- ❑ Royal Order of Scotland
- ❑ Order of Knight Masons
- ❑ Research Lodge
- ❑ Corks
- ❑ Women & Freemasonry
- ❑ International Order of the Rainbow for Girls
- ❑ Job's Daughters
- ❑ DeMolay
- ❑ Co-Freemasonry
- ❑ Order of the Eastern Star
- ❑ Order of Amaranth
- ❑ Knight Kadosh
- ❑ Red Cross of Constantin

Prayer to break unhealthy covenants:

Dear Jesus, I repent of my involvement/I forgive any family members for their involvement with any secret societies that form covenants that affect my family or me. In Your name, Jesus, I break all covenants made by me or by others on my behalf and declare that Your new covenant, which was paid for by your blood, takes precedence over all these other covenants. I reject any curses or blessings associated with these other covenants, and I thank You that You became a curse on my behalf. I confirm that You are the true Source of all spiritual blessings. Amen.

(Note: Some people who have been heavily involved in free-masonry and progressed through a number of ranks, will have made so many covenants that it is sometimes helpful to be more thorough and renounce each covenant separately. I have found the

Freemasonry Release prayer from Jubilee Resources International very useful in this regard.[176])

STEP E: SEXUAL SIN

List all the people you have had sexual encounters with outside of marriage. Ask the Holy Spirit to also highlight any people you have formed unhealthy emotional ties with.

Pray the following prayer for each name listed above.

Jesus, I choose to break all soul ties with _____ and ask that You would cut off all unhealthy influence from

_____.

If you find yourself having difficultly saying the words of the prayer, pause and ask the Holy Spirit to give you help. It may be helpful to have somebody pray with you while you do this process.

If you looked at pornography it can be helpful to pray the following prayer:

Dear Jesus, I choose to break all soul ties with people I have seen while viewing pornography and ask that You would cut off all unhealthy influence from them, and remove all memories of them. Amen.

STEP F: PARTICIPATION IN ABORTION

If you persuaded somebody to have an abortion it may be helpful to pray the following prayer:

Dear Jesus, I acknowledge that my actions led to the killing of an innocent life. Thank You that You died so that I could be forgiven from this. Please, forgive me and wash my conscience clean. Amen.

---

176. See www.jubileeresources.org (accessed 29 May 2015).

If you had an abortion yourself then it may be helpful to pray this prayer:

Dear Jesus, I acknowledge that my actions led to the killing of an innocent life. Thank You that You died so that I could be forgiven from this. Please, will You forgive me for participating in the killing of Your child, and wash my conscience clean. Amen.

STEP F: FREQUENTLY ASKED QUESTIONS

Do I need to contact the person I have broken a soul tie with?

No, but sometimes the person may suddenly make contact with you. It is as though somehow they are aware that the soul tie has been broken, and they try and reestablish the connection. If it was an unhealthy soul tie then I would suggest not to get back in contact.

What if have now married one of the people I have listed as having a sexual encounter with?

If you haven't already, you need to repent for your part in disobeying God and being sexually intimate outside of a life-long marriage covenant. It may be helpful to adjust the prayer and ask God to break an unhelpful soul ties that have formed, but to keep any healthy soul ties.

If I have remarried do I need to break soul ties with my previous spouse?

I would recommend breaking soul ties with anyone who is not your current spouse.

KEY POINTS

1. The presence of fear in our lives can negatively affect our health. This can happen through in-the-moment fear or through failing to deal appropriately with long-term anxieties or phobias.

2. Sexual and spiritual experimentation can have long-term, unseen effects on our health.

3. Allowing God to deal with these issues can bring significant health improvements.

SECTION THREE:

PURSUING HEALING

"Hope is necessary in every condition.
The miseries of poverty, sickness and captivity would,
without this comfort, be insupportable."
—*William Samuel Johnson*
Eighteenth-century American politician

"We are supernaturalists first, not naturalists.
The only reason we feel compelled to accommodate
science is that science says we ought to.
But it is science that should accommodate revelation.
Revelation has been around much longer."
—*Matt Chandler, The Explicit Gospel*
Twenty-first-century pastor and cancer survivor

CHAPTER 9:

IS GOD PRO-DOCTORS?

"It's not the healthy that need a doctor, but the sick."
—*Jesus of Nazareth*

Concluding its eighth and final season in May 2012, *House*, starring Hugh Laurie, was a very successful medical series about a narcissistic, misanthropic, but diagnostically brilliant hospital doctor. It is not one to watch to be spiritually uplifted, but it does give good insight into the increasingly common arguments of the anti-God worldview we find in the West today. In one episode, called "House vs. God," Dr. House, an avowed atheist, looks after a patient who claims to have a supernatural gift of healing. The episode pits House against supernatural healing as House works to disprove its possibility and his diagnostic team keep tally of "victories" for God and "victories" for Dr. House.

Our beliefs and lifestyles probably bear very little resemblance to Dr. House, but many Christians do something similar and pit the wisdom of healthcare professionals against supernatural healing, as if God should take a side. This divide was illustrated very keenly when I was observing at the Church Hospital in Uganda.

(This was the hospital where I witnessed the anencephalic birth detailed in chapter 1.) Originally the hospital was a mission, but by the time I arrived it had been handed over by the missionaries to the local church. There were still some European and American missionaries who did most of the surgery, but there was also a local evangelism team that went around praying with people for their healing. The Christian doctors did their surgery while the Christian pastors prayed with patients—completely separately.

"If we are all Christians, why aren't we all praying for the patients prior to surgery?" I thought one day as I observed an operation. "We'd only have to do surgery if supernatural healing didn't occur." I mused some more. "And why aren't the doctors chatting to the pastoral team saying 'please pray into this or that specific thing?'" As far as I could see, the Christian doctors ran the hospital in a standard secular way while the Christian pastors prayed for the patients as complete outsiders to the medical staff.

This divide between God's medical wisdom and God's supernatural power has a long history. More recently, the divide hasn't been helped by the teaching that to visit a hospital or a healthcare professional demonstrates a lack of faith in God for healing. For example, the American healing evangelist John G. Lake told his followers "you quit fooling with the doctor."[177] Likewise, the British Pentecostal healer, Smith Wigglesworth, eschewed medical aid, as described by historian Jonas Clark:

> A brother with a healing ministry came and was invited home for tea. Polly asked, "What would you think of a man who preaches divine healing, yet he himself uses medical means every day?" "I should say that man did not fully trust the Lord" was the answer. After the meal, Smith Wigglesworth told the brother that he had suffered from hemorrhoids since childhood and used salts every

177. Christian Assemblies International, "John G. Lake—A Man of Faith and Works," https://www.cai.org/bible-studies/john-g-lake-man-faith-and-works (accessed 29 May 2015).

day. They agreed to trust God for healing and, from that time forward, his system functioned naturally without any means whatsoever. After this, Smith Wigglesworth and his wife, Polly made a pledge to God, "From henceforth no medicine, no doctors, no drugs of any kind shall come into our house.".... In the 1930s, an X-ray revealed Smith Wigglesworth was suffering from kidney stones. An immediate operation was necessary to avoid a painful illness and eventual death. "Doctor, the God who made this body is the one who can cure it. No knife shall ever cut it as long as I live" was his response. He endured six years of pain before he was delivered. Later he suffered from sciatica which made walking painful and often, he was more sick than the people he prayed for! At seventy-eight he ruptured badly and in 1944 he suffered a slight stroke.[178]

While I can understand the heart of their sentiments, I don't believe this view is in line with what we read in the Bible, as we shall see through the following accounts.

THE CASE FOR SEEKING HEALING THROUGH MEDICINE AND HEALTHCARE PROFESSIONALS

God seems quite comfortable with people treating illnesses and wounds with medicines. Medicines are mentioned in the Bible directly: *"A joyful heart is good medicine"* (Proverbs 17:22); *"Bruises and sore and raw wounds; they are not pressed out or bound up or softened by oil"* (Isaiah 1:6); *"No medicine for your wound, no healing for you"* (Jeremiah 30:13).

Through the Old Testament laws, God's wisdom for preventing and treating diseases is extensively outlined: the laws taught

178. Jonas Clark, "Smith Wigglesworth: The Apostle of Faith," www.jonasclark. com/revival-history/smith-wigglesworth-the-apostle-faith (accessed 23 April 2015).

the Israelites how to determine which skin diseases were infectious, how to minimize disease spread from dead bodies, how to practice good hygiene, etc.[179]

In the New Testament, we see Jesus affirming the role of the medical profession when He suggested that those who are sick have need of a physician.[180] While His main point was spiritual, for somebody who had an extensive healing ministry, He could have easily decried going to a doctor as a lack of faith—but He didn't. In a similar vein, Jesus commended the Good Samaritan for, among other things, applying ointments to the beaten man's wounds. This practical act of mercy was no doubt part of Jesus' challenge to the religious hearers to *"Go, and do likewise"* (Luke 10:37).

Like Jesus, the apostle Paul didn't seem to see the medical profession as being in opposition to his extensive healing ministry. In his letter to the Colossian church, he casually mentions that *"Luke the beloved physician greets you"* (Colossians 4:14). Luke, who wrote the gospel of Luke and the book of Acts, was one of Paul's closest travelling companions. Paul's warm mention of Luke would hardly have been so warm if Paul thought physicians prevented people from having faith for healing; rather than refer to him by his profession he probably would have referred to him simply as "my travelling companion, Luke." In contrast, having a trained physician travel with Paul was probably extremely helpful because Dr. Luke would have been able to dress Paul's wounds after the many occasions when he was brutally whipped, stoned, and beaten.

On another occasion, rather than advise his colleague Timothy to seek supernatural healing for his frequent stomach upsets, Paul appealed to practical wisdom. In the letter he wrote, he advised Timothy to switch from only drinking untreated water, which commonly contained bugs that caused stomach upsets, to also

---

179. See Leviticus 13:1–59; 15:2–13; Numbers 5:2–4; 19:11–13, 22; Deuteronomy 23:12–13.
180. See Luke 5:31.

drink some wine.[181] The fermentation process of wine is known to kill many of the common bacteria that lead to stomach upsets. For Paul, supernatural healing and medical wisdom were not in opposition to each other.

In the centuries that followed, Christians took an active role in looking after the sick, sometimes risking their lives to look after the victims of plague or other infectious diseases. When Constantine declared the Roman Empire would adopt Christianity, the extensive medical care that was being carried out was formalized. The Church Council of Nicaea in A.D. 325 decided to build a hospital in every town that was big enough to have a cathedral. Bishop Basil of Caesarea (A.D. 329–379) was one of the first to put this into practice. He built a huge hospital, in what is now modern-day Turkey, which had living quarters for doctors and nurses and different areas for different classes of patients. Some of these church-built hospitals had libraries and training programs, and they were the basis for what we know today as a modern in-patient hospital.

So intertwined were hospitals with Christianity around the beginning of the ninth century, the emperor decreed that all hospitals had to be formally attached to either a cathedral or monastery. By the mid-1500s, in just the Benedictine order, there were thirty-seven thousand monasteries that cared for the ill.[182] Unsurprisingly, the old French term for hospital is *hôtel-Dieu*, the "hostel of God."

As time went by, healthcare became more formalized and was often funded privately or by the state, but many Christians were drawn to the health professions and charities because of their faith.

For example, in 1859, Jean-Henri Dunant left his native Switzerland to ask permission from French Emperor Napoléon

---

181. See 1 Timothy 5:23.
182. Brian Barlowe, "Charity and Compassion: Christianity is Good for Culture," September 15, 2008, http://www.probe.org/site/c.fdKEIMNsEoG/b.4496493/k.5E96/Charity_and_Compassion_Christianity_Is_Good_for_Culture (accessed 23 April 2015).

III to do business in French-controlled Algeria. On his visit Jean-Henri found himself witnessing the Battle of Solferino, where forty thousand soldiers died or were wounded. Abandoning his business aspirations completely, for several days he looked after the war-wounded. On his return to Switzerland he co-founded the Red Cross, which has grown into a group of humanitarian organizations with ninety-seven million volunteers, members, and staff worldwide. The Red Cross has won the Nobel Peace Prize three times for its work with war-wounded soldiers and civilians. Jean-Henri confessed, "I am a disciple of Christ as in the first century, and nothing more."[183] For Jean-Henri, caring for the wounds of those injured in war was a natural outworking of his faith.

Joseph Lister (1827–1912) has probably saved the lives of millions of people around the world with his discovery of antiseptic conditions for surgery and post-operative wound healing. In Lister's day, it was still common practice to go from performing an autopsy to carrying out surgery without washing one's hands. As well as introducing phenol to sterilize instruments, he insisted his colleagues wear clean gloves and carry out strict hand-washing procedures. King Edward VII heard of Lister's dramatic success and insisted Lister instruct his surgeon in appropriate antiseptic wound care prior to the king's appendectomy. By following Lister's detailed instructions, the royal surgeon performed a successful operation. Lister had a deep faith and, on one occasion when commissioning newly-qualified doctors, made this charge to them: "It is our proud office to tend the fleshly tabernacle of the immortal spirit, and our path, if rightly followed, will be guided by unfettered truth and love unfeigned. In pursuit of this noble and holy calling I wish you all God-speed."[184]

A more recent example of a doctor whose faith drove all he did is Dr. C. Everett Koop (1916–2013). Dr. Koop had a prolific

---

183. A. J. Schmidt, *How Christianity Changed the World* (Grand Rapids, MI: Zondervan, 2004), 155–66.
184. Time Tracts, "Joseph Lister: God's Surgeon, http://timetracts.com/Home/tracts/heroes-of-the-faith/joseph-lister-gods-surgeon/ (accessed 29 May 2015).

forty-year career in pediatric surgery, pioneering new techniques for conjoined twins and pediatric heart surgery. He said this about the interaction of his faith and work:

> Let me assure you that if I thought that I was walking into that operating room in my own steam, my own power, my own knowledge and was going to operate upon your child—and its survival depended upon me—I wouldn't open the door. I believe that I am a servant of the Lord and that I am going to that operating room with gifts that He has given me. But your child is in His hands, and He will guide me, and I will let you know everything I can about the future of your child.[185]

So respected in his field was Dr. Koop that at age sixty-four he was appointed United States Surgeon General, the most senior doctor of the nation. During his time he helped the nation through the AIDS crisis in the 1980s, and spoke passionately about the dangers of tobacco, leading to twenty million fewer smokers during his eight-year stint. He spoke up about the rights of babies born with birth defects and handicaps and was vocal about his own stance opposing abortion.

I would love to give more examples but space doesn't allow me to mention the many other notable Christian healthcare professionals that made significant discoveries in the area of health, or the thousands, if not tens of thousands of medical missionaries that have travelled overseas to treat people less fortunate than themselves and share the good news of Jesus. And I could only scratch the surface of the millions of Christian doctors, nurses, physios, pharmacists, etc. that, in response to their faith, have chosen to serve God in the healthcare professions.

---

185. Justin Taylor, "C. Everett Koop (1916–2013)," February 25, 2013, http://thegospelcoalition.org/blogs/justintaylor/2013/02/25/c-everett-koop-1916-2013/ (accessed 23 April 2015).

As one of those millions who made that initial choice to work in healthcare, I can say, alongside the prominent characters in the New Testament, that medicine and supernatural healing are not in conflict with each other but are actually complementary. God has gifted healthcare professionals to the world as one of the important ways that He brings healing. However, in going to healthcare professionals we mustn't make the mistake of King Asa: *"In the thirty-ninth year of his reign Asa was diseased in his feet, and his disease became severe. Yet even in his disease he did not seek the Lord, but sought help from physicians"* (2 Chronicles 16:12).

Seeking God for healing is the first thing we must do, and when we do go to healthcare professionals, our trust should be in God, not man. As we seek God for healing, He may direct us to the many great healthcare professionals that have accessed His healing wisdom, but alternatively He might grant us healing through supernatural means.

THE CASE FOR SEEKING SUPERNATURAL HEALING

As we have seen, God is active in healing supernaturally today. In chapter 1 we saw how the twelve, the seventy-two, and then all of us who believe were commissioned to pray for the sick.[186] We then saw how this practice carried on with the apostle Paul, and non-apostles such as Philip and Stephen. In the appendix, I show how the gift of healing has continued throughout every century, and wasn't restricted in use for only during the time of the apostles. In chapter 4, I referenced how the apostle James instructs us to pray for healing after we have confessed sin, and, in chapter 10 we'll go into more detail and look at James's further instructions involving church leaders and the use of oil.

As we have seen, the Bible frequently exhorts Christians to pray for healing, but what about seeking healing ourselves? Does God

---

186. See Matthew 10:1; Luke 10:1–2, 9; Mark 16:17–18.

want us to ask Him for our own supernatural healing? To answer this question, it is helpful to first look at the purpose of healing.

THE PURPOSE OF SUPERNATURAL HEALING

As we saw in chapter 1, supernatural healing represents a foretaste of God's future kingdom, a place where sickness no longer exists. There are four purposes given in the New Testament as to why healing is given to us as this foretaste:

1. It is validation of a divine origin.

When John the Baptist's followers asked Jesus if He was the Messiah, He didn't reason with them or quote the Old Testament prophecies about Himself, but He simply referred them to the healings that had happened through Him: *"The blind receive their sight and the lame walk, lepers are cleansed and the deaf hear, and the dead are raised up, and the poor have good news preached to them"* (Matthew 11:5).

When Jesus' followers also healed people who were sick, they were demonstrating that their ministry also had a divine origin. It wasn't their words that posed a problem for the religious leaders, but rather their healing miracles: *"What shall we do with these men? For that a notable sign has been performed through them is evident to all the inhabitants of Jerusalem, and we cannot deny it"* (Acts 4:16).

So, in Mark chapter 16, when Jesus commissions His disciples (a commission that includes believers today), it is unsurprising this includes the task of praying for the sick. Supernatural healing points to a supernatural origin.

2. It is validation that what Jesus spoke of will come true.

Jesus' declaration that there will be a future resurrection was made more credible by His own resurrection. Likewise, the healing Jesus carried out on earth (and continues to carry out from heaven) gives credibility to Jesus' promise of complete healing when the kingdom is fully ushered in. For instance, by forgiving the paralyzed man and then healing him, Jesus was demonstrating that He had the power to deal both with sin and with its effects.[187]

Before I became a pastor, I was sitting in church one Sunday and felt that God wanted to heal somebody who had a hearing defect in his or her right ear. I mentioned this to the leader of the meeting, and at the end of the service he offered people to come forward for prayer. Three people came forward in response to the request, and I prayed for an older gentleman who had lost his hearing in one ear after a viral ear infection.

I went to place my hand next to his right ear, but he stopped me and explained that the hearing defect was in his left ear. He realized it was not the ear mentioned in the word of knowledge, but he felt he should come forward anyway. I was a little hesitant as my other two colleagues were praying for people with right ear defects, but I decided to pray anyway. Quite wonderfully he and one of the other people being prayed for experienced an instant change in their hearing. I wasn't able to follow up on the other person, but the gentleman I prayed for has full hearing in his left ear to this day. God announced that He wanted to heal, and He backed up His word by healing.

3. It is to point people to God.

The Bible says that supernatural healing is a sign and a wonder. If you drive along a road you will see signs whose purpose is to point you to something. Earthly signs point to earthly things and supernatural signs point to supernatural things. In a similar vein, wonders are things so out of the ordinary that people can't help pondering if there is a realm beyond the natural one. In the New Testament, proclamation of the gospel often went hand-in-hand with supernatural demonstration of the gospel through signs and wonders: *"And awe came upon every soul, and many signs and wonders were being done through the apostles"* (Acts 2:43); *"For I will not venture to speak of anything except what Christ has accomplished through me to bring the*

---

187. See Mark 2:1–12.

Gentiles to obedience—by word and deed, by the power of signs and wonders, by the power of the Spirit of God—so that…I have fulfilled the ministry of the gospel of Christ" (Romans 15:18–19).

Similarly, the gentleman whose ear I prayed for told me he had been struggling with belief in God, but after his healing he was suddenly aware that God wanted to be active in his life. The miracle he received pointed him to God and strengthened his belief.

4. It is a family blessing.

For many years I thought the first three were the only purposes for healing, but more recently I have seen that God has a fourth purpose in healing. Have you ever heard the phrase "family hold back"? When you were a kid and your family had unexpected visitors at a meal, and there is a concern there might not be enough food to go around, you might hear your older brother or mother send the message "family hold back." At a previous church we held an evangelistic event where we were providing food, and it seemed as though we had under-catered. The lead pastor was very concerned that nothing stopped people from staying to hear the great news of the gospel, so he went round to the members of the church giving the same message: family hold back!

It can sometimes feel like God favors those on the edge with experiences of His closeness and healings, but tells those of us already in the family to "hold back." The parable of the lost sheep seems to show that God's bias is to go after the one who is lost and leave the ninety-nine unattended.[188] Likewise, the older brother in the parable of the prodigal son angrily complained, *"you never gave me a young goat, that I might celebrate with my friends. But when this son of yours came, who has devoured your property with prostitutes, you killed the fattened calf for him!"* (Luke 15:29–30).

If this is your experience, or you feel this way, then something isn't quite right. In the prodigal parable, the father replies to the older brother, saying *"Son, you are always with me, and all that is*

---

188. See Matthew 18:12–14.

mine is yours" (verse 31). In effect, "You could have had a goat or a fattened calf at any time you liked." When the shepherd left the ninety-nine sheep it was only briefly, and it was because they were able to be left. The sheep in the flock got the benefit of the shepherd night and day, being fed and tended by him. "Family hold back" only applies when there seems to be a lack, and God has never given us the impression that He is lacking anything.

When the Syrophoenician woman came to Jesus asking for deliverance for her daughter from an evil spirit, Jesus turned the "family hold back" mind-set on its head.[189] As you may know, Jesus did grant her daughter freedom, but not until He had emphasized that this "bread" was primarily for God's children; outsiders received it in second place. For those of us who are one of God's children, then all the benefits of being part of God's kingdom are accessible to us. It's our bread!

The gospel isn't some sales pitch that entices you in, and then, once you have signed, you realize it wasn't as good a deal as you first thought. The gospel really is great news. Part of the great news is guaranteed eternal healing and access to a Father who loves to give His children healing in the here and now. What good earthly father would hold something back from his children, but then give it to children outside of the family? God, who is much better than earthly fathers, certainly wouldn't do such a thing.

While there are an abundance of examples in the Old Testament of God healing His people, have a look at these examples of believers in the New Testament:

+ Paul was healed of a poisonous snake bite.[190]

+ Eutychus was listening to Paul late at night when he fell out of the window and died. Paul ran down and successfully prayed for his resurrection.[191]

---

189. See Matthew 15:22.
190. See Acts 28:3–6.
191. See Acts 20:9–10.

+ Epaphroditus was sick to the point of death but God had *"mercy on him"* (Philippians 2:25–30).

+ Lazarus, along with his sisters, Mary and Martha, was a disciple of Jesus, and Jesus brought him back to life when he died prematurely.[192]

+ Tabitha died from sickness but Peter prayed for her and she came back to life.[193]

God wants us to understand that He is able to cure sickness and He wants us to seek Him for it. Jesus taught us to pray for God's will to be done on earth as it is in heaven. We know what God's heavenly will for sickness is and so we can confidently ask for the same to be carried out here on earth—for us. It wasn't an evangelistic context but a church context when James told us to pray for healing for each other. Likewise in 1 Corinthians, the gift of healing was described as a benefit for the people in the church (for the *"common good"*), in contrast to being a benefit for outsiders: *"To each is given the manifestation of the Spirit for the common good...for to one is given through the Spirit the utterance of wisdom... to another gifts of healing"* (1 Corinthians 12:7–9).

For those of us who believe, while we should always have Jesus' heart for those who are spiritually lost and pray for healing when a situation presents, the gift of healing was also given for the benefit of the church, so we should also pray for each other to be healed.

The Bible teacher and church pastor John Piper, more known for his ministry to the church rather than ministry in evangelism, tells of his experience with the gift of healing:

I don't see any reason that any [of the gifts] should in principle be eliminated from present experience, at least the possibility of God giving it at any time. So I would say, yes there is a gift of healing...the Holy Spirit gives them

192. See John 11.
193. See Acts 9:36–40.

according to His sovereign will...God is sovereign and He is supernatural and He touches and He heals...it is something that goes beyond what doctors can do, though I love doctors...God heals, He heals cancer, He heals sore throats...so we should ask for the gift...I put my hands on people and I ask God then and there to do something... there have been a few where they have come back with excitement that they have been touched and healed.[194]

HOW IS SUPERNATURAL HEALING POSSIBLE?

Healing, like everything a believer experiences, has its root in Jesus' death and resurrection. In Paul's letter to the Romans, we are told that in going to the cross, Jesus became our Substitute.[195] Though He wasn't sick Himself, Matthew tells us that He took on our illnesses and diseases so that we could receive healing: *"He took our illnesses and bore our diseases"* (Matthew 8:17).

As we saw in chapter 1, the fullness of this doesn't happen until Jesus returns and restores all things, but in the meantime this future kingdom sometimes breaks through and we receive healing in this world as well. This is the same for the other things Jesus dealt with through His death and resurrection. For instance, on the cross Jesus bore all our sin,[196] but we will only be fully free from sin when Jesus restores all things. The same is true of curses. Jesus became a curse for us,[197] and while we are free from the curses associated from not fulfilling the law, we are still affected by the curses associated with the fall, such as experiencing difficulty in

---

194. Quoted in Adrian Warnock, "John Piper on Healing," January 30, 2013, http://www.patheos.com/blogs/adrianwarnock/2013/01/john-piper-on-healing/ (accessed 29 May 2015).

195. See Romans 5:8.

196. See 1 Peter 2:24.

197. See Galatians 3:13.

labor and work.[198] On the cross Jesus also triumphed over evil and conquered death, but currently we still experience death and evil.[199] However, when Jesus comes to usher in His kingdom in all its fullness, these will be no more.

What Jesus Achieved			
	At The Cross	**Our Experience Currently**	**The Future Promise**
Sin:	He bore our sin	Experience some freedom	No more sin
Curses:	He became a curse for us	Experience some freedom	No more curses
Sickness:	He bore our sickness	Experience some relief[200]	No more sickness
Death:	He triumphed over death	No fear of death	No more death
Evil:	He triumphed over evil	Increasingly free of evil	No more evil

Some people teach that because Jesus bore our sicknesses, we should receive instant healing every time any sickness comes on us. The argument goes that because forgiveness of sin occurs automatically in response to true repentance, healing from sickness should also be automatic, because they were both achieved through the same thing: Jesus' death and resurrection. When we are sick, it is taught, we should simply pray or claim our healing, and the sickness should leave. The trouble with this argument is that it confuses our individual sins (that create a barrier to God) and the effects of living in a sin-corrupted world (which God only completely deals with when Jesus fully ushers in His kingdom).

198. See Genesis 3:16–19.
199. See Colossians 3:15; Romans 6:9.
200. Through medical intervention or supernatural healing.

The confusion is this: when we repent of sin our relationship with God is restored, but our repentance does not remove the effects of sin from us. For instance, imagine that just as we were repenting to God, somebody tried to steal our watch and broke it in the process. Confessing our sin restores our broken relationship with God but forgiving the perpetrator doesn't restore our broken watch. One of the consequences of living in a sin-corrupted world is that we get sick, and along with decay and death, these consequences of sin only get fully resolved when Jesus returns. Yes, we should pray for healing, but we can't say that because forgiveness from individual sins is fully complete on this side of heaven, our healing should also be fully complete as well. If it were, we should also expect the automatic removal of the other effects of living in a sin-infested world: decay from our body (no aging) and the automatic removal of death from our body (immortality). These results were all achieved through the cross but they have different time periods for us receiving them.

Another way of looking at this is through the journey a believer takes after spiritual rebirth.

The Believer's Journey			
	Born Again	**Life Post-Conversion**	**Kingdom Fully Established**
Salvation:	Declared saved[201]	Working-out of salvation[202]	Salvation fully realized[203]
Deliverance:	Declared delivered[204]	Freedom appropriated through prayer[205]	Fully delivered from evil[206]
Sanctification:	Declared holy[207]	Growing in holiness[208]	Holy as God is holy[209]

The Believer's Journey (cont.)			
	Born Again	**Life Post-Conversion**	**Kingdom Fully Established**
Reconciliation:	Made right with God[210]	Grow in relationship with God[211]	See God face to face[212]
Healing:	Declared healed[213]	May experience some healing[214]	Fully healed[215]

The cross of Calvary is the reason that all the above is even possible. Jesus lived the life we should have lived and died the death that should have been ours, so that we could access all that is His. So the short answer to why supernatural healing is possible is simply the gospel. The gospel offers us a guarantee of complete healing in the future and access to a Father in heaven who loves to give His children a foretaste of healing here on earth. This is gospel-centered healing, and true gospel-centered healing doesn't just focus on the physical but on all of us: spirit, soul, and body.[216]

---

201. See Titus 3:5; Ephesians 2:8.
202. See Philippians 2:12; 1 Corinthians 15:2.
203. See 1 Peter 1:9.
204. See Colossians 1:13.
205. See Matthew 6:13.
206. See Revelation 21:27.
207. See Colossians 3:12; 1 Peter 2:9.
208. See 1 Peter 1:15.
209. See Revelation 21:27.
210. See Romans 5:1.
211. See John 15:15.
212. See Matthew 5:8; 1 Corinthians 13:12; Revelation 22:4.
213. See 1 Peter 2:24.
214. See James 5:16.
215. See Revelation 21:4.
216. See 1 Thessalonians 5:23 and Hebrews 4:12.

Gospel-centered healing			
	Born Again	**Life Post-Conversion**	**Kingdom Fully Established**
Spirit:	Fully healed	Fully healed	Fully healed
Soul (mind, emotions, will):	Some healing	Ongoing healing process	Fully healed
Body:	May experience healing	May experience healing	Fully healed

Once we have been adopted into God's family we can approach our Father in heaven for wisdom on how to receive all sorts of healing; when it comes to bodily sickness, He may direct us to healthcare professionals or prayer for supernatural healing, and He may point us to receive spiritual and emotional healing first.

What sicknesses are present in your body currently? What are the sicknesses in your soul or spirit currently? Have you ever asked God for His wisdom in how to receive healing for each of these and the order He may want you to follow?

KEY POINTS

1. The divide between God's medical wisdom and God's supernatural power has a long history, but it has no foundation in the Bible.

2. Seeking God for healing is the first thing we must do. He may direct us to the many great healthcare professionals that have accessed His healing wisdom, but alternatively He might heal us supernaturally.

3. Supernatural healing has four purposes: It is a validation of a divine origin, it is validation that what Jesus spoke of will come true, it points people to God, and it is a blessing to the family of God.

CHAPTER 10:

REAL *FAITH HEALING*

"He sent out his word and healed them,
and delivered them from their destruction."
— *Jewish Psalmist*

We were sitting in a darkened warehouse and someone came to the microphone and said "God has told me there are three people here who are troubled with backache and the pain is going down one of your legs." My brother and I had just had a great week racing down water slides, competing in sports tournaments, and playing fun adventure games. We were at Spring Harvest, an annual UK Christian conference that, at its peak, gathered seventy thousand people across five resorts during the Easter period. While my parents went to different seminars and teaching events, we participated in the full children's program that was a mixture of fun, games, and Bible teaching.

I was eleven years old and this was the last night of the children's program. After spending some time singing worship songs, my brother and I were a little bemused as we saw, for the first time, people respond in a very un-British way to the presence of the Holy Spirit. It was during this time that the call came out for those with back pain to come forward. As well as having back pain, I had an inner sense that I was one of the people being referred to. I had had back pain for a little while (which, in retrospect, was unusual for a child my age), and the person up front had described the symptoms accurately. I knew I ought to go forward, but a part of me didn't really want to. They made one more call from the microphone asking if the final person could come forward. This was enough of a prompt, and I at long last decided to go. Next to the guy who made the call were two other boys my age. He suggested we sit down, and he explained that he felt our back pain was because we had one leg shorter than the other. He asked if we could pray, and he said a short prayer asking for Jesus to heal our back pain.

Nothing dramatic happened, but I did seem to get some relief from the pain. However, during my teenage years the pain came and went at different periods. Little did I know that God wasn't finished with my back pain, and He was going to do something that would give me the faith needed to help others with the same problem.

I was in my final year of medical school, and our church in Manchester, England, hosted a conference with Terry Virgo as the main speaker. Terry founded the movement our church was a part of and grew it to seven hundred other churches around the world. He had a strong gift of healing, and although on this night he spoke on a message unconnected to healing, at the end of the talk he testified about how he had recently been healed of long-standing back pain. A church leader in India that he knew had sat him down and showed Terry that his legs were different lengths. Following the process I described in chapter 1, Terry watched one of his legs grow supernaturally to the same length as the other. God spoke to Terry and said He wanted him to help others with back pain, and at the time it was Terry's practice to do so wherever he spoke.

After his talk Terry asked if everybody who suffered with back pain could gather and sit in the chairs to the left of the stage, and one by one Terry sat in front of them on the floor and measured their legs. If he found one of their legs to be shorter than the other, he would command the shorter leg, in the name of Jesus, to grow. Rather than sit waiting our turn, my friend James (a qualified physiotherapist) and I stared agog as we saw leg after leg growing. We had never seen anything like this before. When it came to our turn, we were full of faith that God would heal us. Terry showed us how my left leg was one centimeter shorter than my right and how James' right leg was one centimeter shorter than his left. I made sure, as much as I could, that my hips were square and that this difference was not an illusion. But what I couldn't deny was seeing and feeling my leg grow. It took about a second to happen, and I had never seen anything like it in my life. James' leg did the same thing.

After that, James and I went around gathering anybody else that had ever experienced backache and told them to join the line. Some were a little skeptical but everyone whose backache related to differing leg lengths saw their legs grow. Because of the noise that witnessing these miracles generated, others gathered around to see. As faith for healing continued to rise in the room, people with conditions other than backache asked Terry to pray for them, and they were healed as well.

Amazingly, God had highlighted what my problem was a decade or so earlier, but it was only when I understood what needed to happen and grew in faith that I received God's solution.

WHY FAITH IS IMPORTANT IN HEALING

Faith clearly has a huge part to play in supernatural healing. On a number of occasions, both Jesus and the disciples declared that it was people's faith that caused their healing.[217] When the two blind men came to Jesus for healing, He asked them if they believed He could heal them. On hearing their answer He simply said *"according to your faith be it done to you"* (Matthew 9:29). Faith also works the opposite way. Intriguingly, there were times when Jesus said He couldn't do many miracles because of a collective lack of faith in a place.[218] Jesus also asked people to leave rooms prior to Him praying for or commanding healing if He thought they didn't have faith.[219] I think partly why we saw so many healings that day with Terry Virgo was that there was an atmosphere of faith.

While faith is very important in supernatural healing, it is not as straightforward as some would have us believe. For instance, some teach that healing is dependent solely on the faith of the sick person, but this can't be true. For example, there was the occasion when the Roman commander came to Jesus on behalf of his dying servant, and Jesus declared it was the centurion's faith (not the dying servant's) that led to the healing.[220] Likewise, it was the faith of the friends of the paralytic that Jesus responded to, not the paralytic's faith.[221] There were also times when the person being healed couldn't have had faith. Lazarus and Jairus' daughter were both dead when Jesus commanded life to enter them, and it is impossible for a dead person to have faith.[222] Additionally, on both occasions those surrounding Lazarus and Jairus' daughter didn't seem to have faith for healing because they were already in a state of mourning. Only Jesus was certain of the miracle that was about to happen and that their funeral services were not needed.

While faith is intricately connected to healing, what is extremely significant is that failure to receive healing never led Jesus to condemn the sick person for a lack of faith. If you have

---

217. See Matthew 9:29; Mark 5:34; 10:52; Luke 8:50; 17:19; Acts 3:16; 14:9.
218. See Mark 6:1–7.
219. See Matthew 9:23–25.
220. See Matthew 8:5–13.
221. See Matthew 9:2.
222. See John 11:1–44; Luke 8:41–56.

ever been told that you failed to receive healing because of a lack of faith, know that this is not the heart of God! Jesus never condemned people this way. For instance, when the boy with demon-derived epileptic-like symptoms wasn't healed or delivered, Jesus didn't put the blame on the boy but instead pointed to the disciples' lack of faith.[223]

While faith is important in healing, we can't be prescriptive about who needs to have it. On some occasions the sick person had the faith, on others there was an atmosphere of faith, and on other occasions it was the faith of the person doing the praying that led to healing happening.

THE NEED FOR FAITH ALONG WITH CONVENTIONAL THERAPY

Faith isn't just important in supernatural healing. If we don't want to make the mistake of King Asa who trusted his physicians over God,[224] then we need to ensure that as we go to healthcare professionals, we have faith that God can use them to bring about health.

Matt Chandler is one of the most downloaded American preachers on iTunes. He is the lead pastor of The Village Church in Texas and president of Acts 29, a worldwide church-planting network of five hundred plus churches. At the age of twenty-eight he took over the leadership of The Village Church and in a space of twelve years has taken it from one hundred and forty members to over ten thousand. In his own words, up until his thirty-fifth year, life and ministry were "very easy." However, things changed dramatically for him on Thanksgiving morning back in 2009.

He came downstairs, grabbed some coffee, and sat down to feed his six-month-old daughter. The next thing he knew he was

223. See Matthew 17:17–20.
224. See 2 Chronicles 16:12.

lying in hospital. He wasn't aware of losing consciousness, of biting his tongue, or of having a seizure. Neither was he aware of punching the ambulance technician who tried to put a drip in his arm. After various scans, the news quickly came that a piece of abnormal tissue had been found in the frontal lobe of his brain. After making a crescent-shaped incision across half of his skull, his neurosurgeon was able to remove the tissue and a pathologist identified it as a grade three anaplastic oligodendroglioma—a malignant brain cancer. Oligodendrogliomas arise from the supporting tissue in the brain and usually grow in the frontal lobe and present themselves with a seizure around age thirty-five. Matt's experience was typical of the seven hundred and fifty Americans who develop this cancer each year. Classified as grade three, this meant the prognosis of his cancer was not great. At the time, his surgeon told him he should expect to live two to three more years. In an interview given around that time, Matt demonstrated his resolute faith in God in response to this dire prognosis:

> He can heal me. I believe He will. I believe I'm going to be an old surly Baptist preacher. And even if He doesn't... that's the thing: I've read Philippians 1. I know what Paul says. I'm here, let's work. If I go home? That's better. I understand that.

Matt submitted himself to the advice of the medical establishment and took a grueling course of radiotherapy and chemotherapy; people marveled at his faith through the discomfort. Amazingly, after eighteen months of treatment, there is still to this day no sign of the cancer. Matt continues to lead the church that he loves in Flower Mound, Texas. When asked what his advice is to believers who are diagnosed with cancer, he said this:

> I learned very early that people need to have a good grasp of God's goodness and God's sovereignty. On the day that a person is diagnosed, I try to encourage them in God's knowledge—that this hasn't surprised Him or

caught Him off guard. I want to remind them that this isn't punitive, but rather that God is on the move and He can be trusted. Six months after the diagnosis is harder to answer because cancer can go one of two ways. If the man or woman is still in a real fight, I want to draw his or her attention to Hebrews 11 or the story of Abraham being promised a son or even David being anointed king and then running from Saul for all those years before sitting on the throne. I think it's important to remind people after the initial shock of diagnosis wears off and the wear and tear of treatment settles in, that victory, for those who are children of God, is guaranteed, although difficulty, pain, and waiting might all be very present.[225]

In short he encourages people to persist in faith during their illness. But what exactly *is* faith, and more specifically, what is it to have faith for healing?

DEFINING FAITH

Jesus considers faith to be a precious commodity. He *"marveled"* (Luke 7:9) at the centurion's faith and was shocked at His home village's *"lack of faith"* (Mark 6:6 NIV). He asked His disciples if He would find faith on the earth when He returned and prayed that Satan wouldn't take away Peter's faith.[226] Once he had ascended, he appeared to John and told him to tell the Thyatira church that He knew their faith[227] and commended the Pergamum church for not hiding their faith.[228]

Following on from Jesus, Peter told the churches under his care that faith has a greater value than gold. He went on to say

---

225. Matt Chandler, "Don't Waste Your Cancer: Interview with Matt Chandler, *Tabletalk*, July 1, 2011, http://www.ligonier.org/learn/articles/dont-waste-your-cancer-interview-matt-chandler/ (accessed 29 May 2015).

226. See Luke 18:8; 22:32.

227. See Revelation 2:19

228. See Revelation 2:13.

that this precious commodity[229] is needed to resist the devil.[230] In a similar vein, Paul tells us we need faith to resist sin.[231] Finally, the writer to the Hebrews puts it bluntly, saying that faith is one of the elementary teachings, and without faith it is impossible *to please God.*[232]

As you can see, faith clearly is an important part of living the Christian life. People even refer to Christians as "people of faith" or they may say, "I wish I had their faith." But while many people acknowledge faith's importance, they cannot always give a good definition of it.

Fortunately the writer to the Hebrews leaves us in no doubt of what faith is: *"Now faith is the assurance of things hoped for, the conviction of things not seen"* (Hebrews 11:1).

This definition tells us a number of things.

First, faith is not abstract but something tangible. Other translations state that faith is the substance of things hoped for. Faith is substantial. Hebrews 11:6 tells us that faith is something that can be tested, and at times both Jesus and Paul "saw" people's faith (Matthew 9:2; Acts 14:9).

Second, faith leads to action. If faith is a conviction then you would expect people to act on that conviction. For example, when the friends of a paralytic man took time and effort to carry him to Jesus (even breaking down part of a house to gain access) it is recorded that Jesus saw their faith.[233] They wouldn't have done all that if they didn't think there was a chance that Jesus could heal him. They had a *hope* that their friend could be healed, but then acting in faith they made sure that their paralytic friend was placed in front of Jesus.

---

229. See 1 Peter 1:7.
230. See 1 Peter 5:7–9.
231. See Romans 14:23.
232. See Hebrews 6:1; 11:6.
233. See Mark 2:3.

Third, faith is only needed when you don't see the outcome. Faith is the assurance of things unseen, not seen. Once you can see whatever you are standing in faith for, then faith has done its job and you no longer need it. To live by faith is to act from the knowledge that something not yet visible is occurring, or will occur.

We act in faith all the time. Getting on a plane requires a lot of faith. The only thing that keeps that huge volume of metal up in the air is upward force that is generated when air passes at a high speed over its curved wings. Nobody has seen this upward force, but when we step on the plane we act confidently, expecting this force to be generated and, more importantly, maintained. Every moment we live is lived in faith. Likewise, while all of us have learned at some point about the gas essential to life, oxygen, I doubt that anybody has actually seen a molecule of it. I haven't seen one but every second of the day, in faith, I breathe in air trusting that it contains enough oxygen to nourish my tissues.

So you can see that in a broad sense all of us have faith. But biblical faith has a very specific object: God.[234] It's easy to have faith in something explainable and comprehensible, like the physics that allow a plane to take off, but it's a lot harder to have faith in the Creator of the universe.

Some people find it too hard, and instead take their faith off of God and put it fully on a new treatment or a new specialist but this can be dangerous: people and things often let us down, but God never will. Some feel that they just don't have enough faith, but they do not realize that it is not primarily the amount of faith that matters, but where their faith is directed. If it is in the right place, it can quickly grow.

To illustrate faith, Tim Keller tells a story of two rock climbers on a cliff face thousands of feet above sea level. Imagine that the climbers have reached a stage where they can only progress forward if they let go of the rock they are on and leap to a different

---

234. See Mark 11:22; Acts 3:16; 20:21; 24:24; 26:18; 27:25; and 1 Peter 1:21.

foothold. The first rock climber is absolutely certain that the foothold he spies will take his body weight, and he jumps—but the foothold gives way. The second rock climber isn't really sure that the foothold he sees will take his weight but jumps anyway—and it holds firm. Which had the greater faith?

The first rock climber had greater faith in his foothold, but the object of his faith was wrong. The second rock climber had only a small amount of faith that his foothold would hold but because he put it in the right object, he didn't fall. If we place our faith in Jesus, He is a sure Rock that won't give way. Money, popularity, friendship may give way but Jesus won't. Jesus said that if He is the object of our faith, then with faith the size of a mustard seed we might move mountains.[235]

So when it comes to faith, the first thing to check is that the object of our faith is Jesus. Faith in friends, formulas, or feelings, isn't helpful. Jesus is the only one who has the power to act so our faith needs to be in Him. And it is important to remember that Jesus is a Person. He is not some cosmic slot machine that gives out healing if you insert the right prayer. When He healed on earth it wasn't the case of somebody speaking the correct sequence of words to obtain their healing. He always treated people according to their individual situation. You can't form a standardized methodology from the way Jesus acted because He healed many people in many different ways. There are certainly principles that we can learn, and I will look at these later, but Jesus always treated people case by case, according to their faith. Once we realize that Jesus needs to be the object of our faith, we must grow our faith by coming to Him and discover what He is saying about our situation.

Just before our first child was born, the place where I worked was restructuring, and I was laid off. The timing couldn't have been worse. I was shaken up after meeting with my boss, but I walked away and found a quiet place and connected with God.

---

235. See Matthew 17:20.

I spent time worshipping Him and telling Him of my concerns. The time lasted an hour, but at the end of it I felt God's peace. He assured me He was in this layoff and that He had a plan. My wife Michelle and I used the time to brainstorm the options. Was God moving us away from Johannesburg? Or even away from South Africa? When we prayed, I felt God state that He had a church for us locally that would offer me a job.

I followed what God told me to do, but people got nervous on my behalf and felt I should be doing more. Ten years earlier things would have been quite different, and I would have joined them, but that's why section two of this book (chapters 5 through 8) is very important. We need to remove blockages to God so that we can have true biblical faith, and learn to trust Him in situations such as mine. True to His word, God came through exactly as He said He would and provided a job for me locally, and I didn't even miss a single salary payment.

FAITH IN A PERSON

Forgetting that faith needs to be in a Person is one of the common reasons our faith for healing can be faulty. We disconnect from God as a Person and base our faith in other things. In our sickness we need to go to God and find His will and plan. The trouble is that we can be so caught up in the need for physical healing that we can miss the place where God desires to start healing us. Or we can be so focused on people who pray for us, or the voice of healthcare professionals, that we miss God's voice.

Well-wishers, often with good intentions, may make unhelpful statements and pronouncements about God, when what we actually need is God Himself. The story of Job illustrates this situation only too well; in a time of disaster, Job's friends made long and lofty speeches about the cause of Job's calamities and sickness, but their claims were later found to be false. The need for God's voice during sickness is real; without it, and the hope He gives, you can find yourself inwardly groaning when somebody wants to pray for physical healing—yet again, even after years of being sick. If this has happened to you, you may find it wise to increase your faith, before you give consent for people to pray with you.

CAN WE INCREASE OUR FAITH?

While bad experiences, fatigue, and disconnection from God are big sources of weakened faith for healing, our faith is also influenced by the situation surrounding us in the worldwide church. In general, the global church is still journeying to recover the faith pattern set by the early church for supernatural healing. In recent centuries, we have seen an encouraging growth of faith in the worldwide church, in a number of areas, and it is my belief that we are on an upward growth curve of increasing healings. Those of us looking to God for healing can benefit from this growth curve. Let me explain.

FAITH FOR SALVATION ASSURANCE

In Europe during the Middle Ages, there wasn't a good understanding about how to be saved apart from works. The dominant church at that time taught that salvation was dependent on a mixture of faith *and* good works. While the Bible is clear that faith should not remain devoid of good works,[236] good works are explicitly said to follow saving faith rather than being a prerequisite to salvation.[237] For example, if my wife, Michelle, and I were to adopt a child, we wouldn't base our adoption on the child's good behavior, but once we had adopted him or her, as part of Butterworth family life, we would teach and train good behavior.

The fruit of the faulty teaching that salvation depended on works threw believers into great fear over whether they'd end up in heaven when they died. Few understood what it meant to live in God's grace as God's child while on earth. Martin Luther and

---

236. See James 2:19–20.
237. See Romans 3:28 and Galatians 2:16.

John Calvin were pivotal in correcting this misunderstanding, and almost five hundred years later we can bask in the widespread result of their reformative work, living with assurance of our place in heaven, our adoption into God's family, and all the benefits that brings. Because of this, it is much easier for us to have faith for assurance of salvation than it was for our counterparts five hundred years earlier.

FAITH FOR WORLD MISSION

In the eighteenth century, the worldwide church was predominantly pastoral, and Jesus' Great Commission to preach the gospel to the ends of the earth was deemphasized because few had the faith to embrace it. The pattern that Paul established of travelling to other countries to preach the good news had largely been lost.

However, Jesus placed the urge strongly on a young Baptist minister named William Carey to go overseas and preach the gospel. At a ministers' meeting in England in 1786, he asked whether it was the duty of all Christians to spread the gospel throughout the world. His older colleague, John Collett Ryland, is reported to have responded saying: "Young man, sit down; when God pleases to convert the heathen, He will do it without your aid and mine."

Ignoring that discouragement, and acting on his conviction, six years later William Carey founded the Baptist Missionary Society (now called BMS), an organization that over two hundred and twenty years later is still active and currently supports three hundred and fifty missionaries in forty countries. Carey, its first missionary, was sent to Bengal, India, in 1793, where he translated the Bible into Bengali and later Sanskrit. During his lifetime, the mission would go on to translate the Bible, in whole or in part, into a further forty-four languages. Carey spent forty-one years in India and saw seven hundred converts, but his greatest legacy was raising faith in the church for world missions. At the time of Carey's trip there were estimated to be only a few hundred protestant missionaries in the world, but by 1900, this number had grown to fifteen thousand. Thanks largely to Carey's vision and the efforts of these men and women, 67 percent of all active protestant Christians live in countries that were evangelized by missionaries from the last two centuries.[238]

FAITH FOR GIFTS OF THE SPIRIT

Prior to the twentieth century, faith for asking God for supernatural gifts (such as healing) was not common in the worldwide church. However, in 1906, Pentecostalism was born, followed by the Charismatic movement in the 1960s, which brought the practicing of the more supernatural spiritual gifts into the traditional denominations. Because of these two movements, the worldwide church is experiencing many of the supernatural gifts that the New Testament church experienced, and continuationism, the belief that spiritual gifts continue to this day, is the majority belief in the worldwide church. Over the course of a century, faith for supernatural gifts in the worldwide church has dramatically changed.

FAITH FOR HEALING

In response to the growing belief that all the gifts of the Spirit are available to the church today, healing and prayers for healing have started to once again be a normal aspect of church life, at least in some churches. The more success the church sees, the more likely it is that people will have faith to ask God for healing and so forth. As faith for healing collectively grows, it will be easier to have individual faith for healing.

HOW TO INCREASE YOUR FAITH

While we only play a small part in the worldwide church's collective faith for healing, the good news is that once we have faith

---

238. See Paul E. Pierson, "Why Did the 1800s Explode with Missions?" *Christianity Today*, October 1, 1992, http://www.christianitytoday.com/ch/1992/issue36/3620.html (accessed 29 May 2015).

in the right place, we can go on to increase our faith. Paul, in his letter to the Romans, tells us that faith can be held in differing proportions, but he also tells us that faith can grow and increase to the point where we can excel in faith and, as Luke tells us, be full of it.[239]

How would you rate your faith at the moment? Has there been a time in your life when you were full of faith? When in your life have you felt weakest in faith? Whatever levels of faith you feel you have currently, it may be helpful to consider six ways that you can increase in biblical faith.

1. Get the right view of God.

The centurion had faith that Jesus marveled over because he understood correctly the authority Jesus had.[240] If we are going to have faith for healing (at whatever level: body, spirit, or soul), we have to believe that God is able and willing to heal us, regardless of whether He uses supernatural or conventional means. Section two of the book was designed for this purpose: to identify and remove blockages between God and us.

2. Hear from God.

Because faith starts in a person, the way we get faith is by going to God and hearing what He wants to say about our situation: *"Faith comes from hearing..."* (Romans 10:17). In any area where we are deeply involved, it can be difficult to always hear what God is saying, but listen to what that Romans verse goes on to say: *"...and hearing through the word of Christ."* The easiest way to hear from God is to read what He has already said. As we read the Bible, asking God to speak to us, often the Holy Spirit will quicken certain words or phrases that are relevant to our situation.

God also speaks through other people. As I have gotten older I have learned to recognize when a piece of wisdom spoken by

---

239. See Romans 12:6; 2 Thessalonians 1:3; 2 Corinthians 8:7; 10:15; and Acts 6:5; 11:24.
240. See Matthew 8:5–10.

somebody really stands out. I have learned to pray, "Is this You speaking through this person, Lord?" If we surround ourselves with people who have a close walk with God, then it is more likely that God's wisdom is going to overflow from them to us.

God also speaks directly to our minds. Jesus said, "*My sheep hear my voice*" (John 10:27). These last two ways God speaks are more subjective, so we must always weigh what we perceive to be the voice of God against what we already know of God. If God is speaking it is important to remember that He will never contradict what He has already spoken in His Word, the Bible.

There are a few common things that God will say to your heart. First, He often tells you to be part of a healthy church. Other people's faith can rub off on us if we are around them long enough to be encouraged by them and hear their testimonies. Faith is something others can hear about.[241] If faith comes through hearing, then hearing about other people's faith builds faith.

Second, He often tells His children to look at Him, not at the problem. The Israelites looked up at the bronze snake for healing.[242] They couldn't focus on their symptoms simultaneously. Likewise, Abraham looked at his body as good as dead but then took his eyes off his body and looked to God for the solution.[243]

As you try to discern what God is saying, keep your mind open to the fact that God's priority might be very different from yours. For example Paul said that "*outwardly we are wasting away, yet inwardly we are being renewed day by day*" (2 Corinthians 4:16 NIV), indicating that an inner work was happening despite a bodily decay. And as we have seen in the previous chapters, often physical healing proceeds from an inner work.

3. Bring these words into our heart.

---

241. See Colossians 1:4.
242. See Numbers 21:8.
243. See Hebrews 11:12.

God's words are like seed, and to bear fruit, they need to be planted in our heart. Proverbs tell us, *"Be attentive to my words… keep them within your heart. For they are life to all those who find them, and healing to all their flesh"* (Proverbs 4:20–22). According to this proverb, the healing of our flesh comes from keeping God's words in our heart. When the angel spoke to Mary foretelling the birth of Jesus, Luke tells us that she treasured these words in her heart. We don't all get visitations from angels, but we can all learn to treasure God's Word in the right place. When we do so, it works inside of us and creates faith to act according to God's will.[244]

4. Act on what God says.

Because faith results in action we need to be obedient to whatever we feel God say. Smith Wigglesworth put it succinctly: "First, read the Word of God. Second, consume the Word of God until it consumes you. Third, believe the Word of God. Fourth, act on the Word." [245] If we acknowledge that God really is our Creator and Savior, then we need to honor that and do as He says. If you know the story of Namaan, you'll recollect that he almost didn't receive his healing because he didn't want to carry out the instructions that God gave him.[246]

5. Persist.

Faith receives the promise but patience inherits it: *"Imitate those who through faith and patience inherit what has been promised"* (Hebrews 6:12 NIV). I am not saying you are going to win every battle. Paul saw many healed and even people raised from the dead, but he also unashamedly left Trophimas sick in Melitus.[247] However, I am saying that it is important that we battle. Sickness wasn't God's intention and through Jesus we have access to His wisdom and power to heal. So because of this, it means we should

---

244. See 1 Thessalonians 2:13.
245. Quoted in G. D. Johnson, *What Will a Man Give In Exchange for His Soul?* (Philadelphia, PA: Light of the Savior Ministries, 2011), 119.
246. See 2 Kings 5:9–14.
247. See 2 Timothy 4:19–20.

press into God for healing in our body, soul and spirit, so that every moment of our lives can be lived to their fullest for God's glory.

6. Ask for faith.

God offers faith to us as a gift.[248] When we acknowledge that our faith is low, we can ask Him to give us faith knowing that it is available to us. The father of the epileptic boy who was brought to Jesus said, *"I believe, help my unbelief!"* (Mark 9:24). Jesus didn't seem to mind his honesty and went on to heal his son. It can be difficult to have faith at times, but this is why God provides us with it as a gift.

Where is your faith currently? What things can do you right now to grow your faith? Why not spend a moment putting this into action.

KEY POINTS

1. While faith is intricately connected to healing, the failure to receive healing never led Jesus to condemn the sick person for a lack of faith.

2. We can have faith in many things, but biblical faith relates only to faith in God.

3. We can increase our faith by getting the right view of God, hearing from God, bringing His Word into our hearts, acting on what God says, persisting in those actions, and always asking God for faith.

---

248. See 1 Corinthians 12:9.

CHAPTER 11:

PRAYING FOR DIVINE INTERVENTION

"You will argue with yourself that there is no way forward. But with God, nothing is impossible. He has more ropes and ladders and tunnels out of pits than you can conceive. Wait. Pray without ceasing. Hope."
—*John Piper*
Author, pastor, and cancer survivor

I had a vision of you surrounded by people holding a copy of your book. They were telling you that through reading it, God had healed them."

I was twenty-two years old and I don't think I had even considered writing a book, let alone one on healing. To say I was taken aback by this message was an understatement.

Moments earlier, the pastor who was now telling me about God's intention had just introduced himself. We hadn't met before, but God had seemed to have shown him a vision of what He wanted to do through me in the future. I went away imagining how it might happen, and over the years I treasured it in my heart. I knew that when the time was right, God would lead me to start writing, but at twenty-two years of age I knew I would have to experience people being healed before I could write credibly. Ten years later, I felt God give me the nudge that it was time to start writing.

So, if you are reading these words, then it is important to know that many years ago God declared that He would use this book to heal people. My prayer is that, through following the principles ahead, you will be given the wisdom from God needed to access healing. You may find healing through the right healthcare professional, or you may be surprised by God healing you supernaturally.

I have ordered the biblical principles for praying for healing in a step-wise process that begins with seeking God by yourself and gradually brings others in to pray for you, as the need may arise. As I have stressed before, we need to have confidence in God rather than methods, but I needed to present the principles in an order, and the following seems the most logical one to me. I would encourage that even if you have received lots of prayer by many people, it is still worth working through the process.

PRAYER BY YOURSELF

If you read through the New Testament, you will notice that Jesus did not heal everyone around Him, nor did He seem to go out in search of people to heal. Rather, the people who did receive healing were those who came to Him and interacted with Him. Now that Jesus has ascended to heaven, it is through prayer that we come to Him. Learning to do this successfully is an important principle in seeking healing.

How are you at spending time with God? Do you practice the spiritual disciplines, such as studying the Bible, prayer, and personal worship? Have you learned what it means, as the psalmist says, to wait on God?[249] At some points in my life I have found

---

249. See Psalm 25:5; 37:7, 34; and 62:1.

it quite easy to connect with God, and at other times, it has been quite difficult. It is during those difficult times that I have learned to push through and wait for God. God is willing to interact with us if we would take the time to do so. This isn't a passive waiting, though; it is an active waiting—waiting with an anticipation of a meeting. During my time in Ghana, I stayed with a Korean missionary who took me to a mountain that had been set aside for prayer. I walked into this large wooden hall and I was told that I should pray, and I would be picked up in four hours. Not really knowing what else to do, I knelt down and said, "God, I am with You solely for the next four hours, what would You like us to do?" Quite remarkably, God filled those four hours so that they passed quickly. I was led to read parts of the Bible, to pray for certain people, etc., and I felt God say to me that if I give Him a dedicated time, He will always have a plan for what to do.

When I read the Bible I have found it helpful to ask God, "What do You want to say to me?" As I start to read I am also waiting for God to bring an answer to my question. He may do so by highlighting certain phrases that then resonate with me, or He may cause me to have a new perspective on a passage, which increases my awareness of Him and what He wants to achieve through my life.

As we pray, it is important to ask God questions: "Lord, is this an illness that You want to heal me of while on earth?" "If so, do You want to do it through conventional or supernatural means?" "What is the next step that I must take?" Sometimes when I ask God questions, I get the answer straightaway, and this is often true when I ask Him questions, such as, "What should I do now?" However, there are many occasions when the answer comes later, and in a variety of ways. I feel it is my job to ask God questions and then let Him give the answer in whatever means and timing He may see fit to bring it.

For example, God spoke to me while I was in my second year of university, that I would live in Africa long-term. In response to that, I applied for a short-term mission trip to Uganda later that summer, and then, three years later, I arranged for my three-month elective program to be at a Ghanaian hospital. However, three years after graduating, I was still working in the UK and I remember asking God how I should go about moving out there. A little while later I was browsing the Internet when I came across a scholarship program to do a master's program at the university I had just graduated from. What was interesting is that the master's program had just been converted to be entirely web-based, so it could be done from anywhere in the world. I felt God nudge me to apply; I got the scholarship, and very quickly I was making plans to volunteer for a day or two a week at a church in South Africa that I had several links with. I came out for a year initially, but God opened a door to stay longer. I met my wife and started a family here in South Africa, and I remain in South Africa to this day.

Being obedient to what we think God is saying is important, because we can see that, many times in the Bible, healings did not happen until the person responded in obedience to what Jesus had commanded. For instance, the ten lepers received their healing "*as they went*" to the priests (Luke 17:11–14). The man with the shriveled hand received his healing as he obeyed Jesus to stretch out his hand.[250] A blind man who came to Jesus received his sight as he obeyed Jesus' command to "*wash in the pool of Siloam*" (John 9:1–7).

If we are to live with Jesus being our Lord as well as our Savior, then one of the reasons we pray is so that we understand what He wants us to do. Our job is then to do it.

WHAT SHOULD WE DO WHEN IT SEEMS THAT GOD IS NOT SPEAKING?

This is all very well if you feel you have heard God, but what if it seems as though God is not communicating anything to you? A

---

250. See Matthew 12:9–13.

good place to start is to go back to the last thing He told you and ensure you are obeying that. I have found that God will frequently use silence to bring an unheeded request to our attention. Second, if you are not sure what God wants you to do, I would suggest that you start by doing what is in your power to do. For instance, if you are in a country where malaria is common and you think you have contracted it, then it would be appropriate to go to a doctor to have this confirmed and receive anti-malarial medication. If God has provided you access to a doctor and medication, and the money to pay for it, then it would seem reasonable that God is directing you to receive healing from malaria through anti-malarial medication.

When we are sick, visiting a healthcare professional and getting a diagnosis is important so that we can know exactly what we want God to heal us of. In the book of Genesis, God told Abraham that He was going to give his barren wife, Sarah, a child. The book of Hebrews tells us that Abraham's body was *"as good as dead"* (Hebrews 11:12). He had tried naturally to father a child with Sarah, but he got the diagnosis and realized that he needed a miracle. When we have done our part and reached the end of our resources, then we're in a great place to plead for God's healing grace.

The only time I have broken a bone in my body was when I broke my big toe. I was playing sports and had a chance to score when I clashed with an opponent and landed in an odd way; the force of my whole body landed on the weight of the one toe, causing the bone to fracture. The toe swelled up like a balloon, and I went to the hospital for an X-ray. When the specialist saw me, he told me the fracture had gone into the joint, replacing the joint's smooth surface with a step, where one part of the bone was higher than the other. He predicted that as the toe bone healed, the joint would fuse or at best become arthritic, and I would lose the ability to bend my big toe. I wasn't very pleased at this prospect but the only alternative was private, expensive surgery.

As I was weighing the pros and cons of surgery, I went away for the weekend with some friends. That Sunday we went to a local church in the area where the senior pastor was known to have a gift of healing. After the service my friend and I talked with him and asked him to pray for healing. I was hoping for a dramatic miracle. He prayed a simple prayer asking God for full restoration of the joint, but nothing seemed to happen. Later that evening, I took off my toe's support to have a bath. While I was getting out of the bath, I slipped and reflexively used my injured foot to stop myself from falling. I thought I was about to damage my toe further, but as my weight pressed on the toe, I felt the two parts of the bone slide against each other, seeming to align against the joint. Instead of pain, I could now gently move my joint. The bone healed without the joint fusing, and I can move my big toe just fine to this day, free of arthritis. So in a very unexpected and surprising way, God intervened and answered the pastor's prayer.

If you know the story of Abraham, you'll know that it wasn't as straightforward as Abraham waiting for God to open up Sarah's womb. Prior to the miracle, and perhaps out of the frustration of waiting a long time, Abraham tried to make God's plan happen naturally. I can have some empathy with the situation. God had said that Abraham was going to have a child, but He didn't seem to be keeping that promise! A decade went by. Probably impatient by this time, and following both the pattern of the culture of the day and the suggestion of his wife, he lay with Sarah's maidservant, Hagar, and fathered a son.[251]

To those of us who have grown up with a Christian-based view of marriage, this behavior may seem extremely strange, but Abraham hadn't grown up following God.[252] His father's name, Terah, means "priest," indicating that he was a priest in the ancient city of Ur,[253] where the moon was worshipped. With only his cul-

---

251. See Genesis 16:1–3.
252. See Joshua 24:2.
253. See Genesis 11:27–29.

ture to go on and God's words to him, Abraham probably didn't have the strong theology on covenant marriage that we have today. However, this doesn't detract from the fact that his choice wasn't wise. This wasn't the way God wanted to fulfill His promise. As Christians, like Abraham, we may be tempted to try and make our own plan contrary to God's instruction, even with the full support of our family and culture, but this isn't acting in faith. Faith is not only expressed through asking God *what* He wants to do, but also by asking how He wants to do it. If God has spoken the how, we continue in faith by sticking to it—even if years go by without anything happening.

As we have seen in chapter 8, the rise of alternative belief systems have brought with them many potentially enticing ways to make our own plan for healing. We may even justify it by saying that God has spoken that He wants to heal us, but if God is going to heal, He will do it through ways that do not endanger us spiritually. Chapter 8 has looked at some of the spiritually dangerous healing options, and we should certainly avoid those, but what about the many spiritually neutral alternative medicines and practices that are available nowadays?

When it comes to seeking God for healing through conventional means, it is important to ensure that we really are tapping into God's wisdom. Jesus said that we would know a false prophet by his fruit; or, in other words, by his results.[254] If he were really speaking God's words, then it would come to pass. Likewise, if it really is God's healing wisdom, it will bring results. Mainstream healthcare hasn't always been good at ensuring this, but things are starting to change. Rather than rely on the opinions of eminent experts, healthcare is starting to determine what the wisest approach is through the robust evidence of results. A good example of this evidence-based approach is in the treatment of childhood cancer.

---

254. See Matthew 7:15–16.

In European industrial countries, deaths from almost all childhood cancers have been declining. Between the periods of 1978–1982 to 1993–1997, survival rates have increased by 30 to 50 percent and continue to improve.[255] This massive rise in survival is due to highly standardized and very effective therapeutic regimes that have been agreed upon by cancer experts across many countries. No longer does one pediatric oncologist try one combination of treatment while at another hospital down the road another pediatric oncologist tries a different combination. Each cancer type has specific regimes and massive sets of data are collected to trace the effectiveness. Every so often the regimes are adjusted (as new drugs come to the market) and checked against the data to ensure that the adjustment actually brings improvement in cancer survival. This highly scientific approach has required a lot of coordination and has required oncologists to give up a lot of their previous freedom, but the result has been thousands more cancer survivors. As the regimes are tweaked, survival rates get better all the time.

When seeking healing you should ensure that you apply a similar rigor when deciding the best diagnostic and treatment options. Mainstream healthcare is becoming more and more evidence-based, but a lot of the alternative healthcare options are behind on this. This topic is so large that it goes beyond the scope of this book, but a reliable place to start for evidence searching is the Cochrane Collaboration. This organization gathers the available evidence on a particular topic and combines all the results, in what is called a meta-analysis, and then gives a simple, plain English summary. They have a great search feature for this topic.[256]

This and other evidence searches will only tell you if a particular treatment seems to produce scientifically verifiable results. On top of this, every Christian still needs to apply wisdom to weigh the ethical and spiritual aspects of any potential treatment.

---

255. See K. Pritchard-Jones, et al., "Cancer in children and adolescents in Europe: developments over twenty years and future challenges," *European Journal of Cancer* 42 (2006): 2183–2190.
256. See http://summaries.cochrane.org/search.

Assuming you have obeyed what you feel you need to have obeyed and that you have done your part in seeking healing (in the ways open to you), then you are probably in a good place to ask, also, for supernatural healing. Before you pray I'd suggest you start by building your faith through reminding yourself what Jesus has said about healing: We have access to healing because Jesus bore our sicknesses on the cross,[257] if you are God's child, healing is your *"bread"* (Matthew 15:26), and if you are of Jesus' disciples, you have been given authority over sickness.[258]

Knowing the authority we have been given is an important part of praying for healing. Praying for healing isn't about asking but rather commanding. There isn't a single example in the New Testament where Jesus taught us to ask for healing. Rather, healing is declared, and sickness commanded to leave.

So, if you want to pray for sickness, you need pray from a place of authority and command. When I pray, I command sickness to leave and tell the joints, ligaments, etc., to align themselves with how Jesus wants them to be. An evangelist I know decided to step out in this, and he taught people at big meetings to place hands on sick areas of their bodies and command healing. As he and others stepped into the authority that Jesus has given His disciples, he saw many healings.

Why not try this now? Place a hand over a sick part of your body and, in the name of Jesus, command the sickness to leave. If you felt something change, then, if at all possible, try and test if you have been healed. For example if you couldn't move a joint before, try (gently) to move it.

Something may happen as you pray, but at other times it may not. Once you have commanded take a moment to listen to what God may be saying. You may get a sense of something that needs to be done before God initiates a healing. You should test what

257. See Matthew 8:17.
258. See Mark 16:18.

you sense against the Bible, but if it seems like the sort of thing God would say then it is important to try and be obedient to it. Other times you may not sense anything and, like the instance of my damaged toe joint, sometimes God will intervene as you go about the course of your daily lives.

Once you have prayed alone, if you do not receive healing I would advise you move on to the next step and to seek prayer from others. We are in a battle, and sometimes it can be helpful to fight the battle with some other soldiers.

PRAYER BY OTHER CHRISTIANS

In Mark 16 we see Jesus telling His followers that they will lay hands on the sick and the sick will recover. If you are the one who is sick, and you have Christian friends, it is only reasonable that in accordance with Mark 16, you can ask them to come and lay hands on you and command sickness to leave. I am not talking about people coming to offer healing, but rather you specifically inviting people whom you trust and are comfortable with.

As we will see with Chris's story in chapter 12, if you are sick, many well-meaning people may come to you with all sorts of advice and methodologies to receive healing, and it can often be wise to have somebody filter these ideas. Chris's solution to this was to arrange for anybody who wanted to suggest a special fasting regime or a certain healthcare professional to first speak to one of his fellow pastors. His other pastors would assess whether they thought the advice would be helpful or not. If it was helpful they would be the ones to pass it on. This gave Chris and his family some protection from dealing with the emotional weight of many well-wishers that are often present if you are part of a large church.

It is different, though, when choosing friends to pray for you. Most people want the prayers of their close, believing friends, because prayer is powerful. We saw in chapter 10 that faith is an important part of healing; so when you choose friends to pray for you, it would be wise to ask friends who you know are full of faith. Prayer for healing can become disillusioning if you are prayed for by people who pray out of a sense of duty, or by people who have unhelpful theologies.

If you have been sick for a long time, you may have received lots of prayer and reached a sort of prayer fatigue. Your hopes may have been raised every time a person or group prays, only to be dashed if nothing happens. But this isn't how it is meant to be. With the right people praying, prayer should be a blessing, regardless of the outcome, because it connects you to God. God places us in community and family so that we can support each other. Perhaps when people pray they will get insight into a spiritual condition that could be blocking healing, or they may receive some wisdom to approach a certain healthcare professional that could open up the correct diagnosis or treatment (as we saw through Amy's story in chapter 1).

When it comes to healing, the support of friends can be essential, as the paralyzed man who was carried to Jesus realized.[259] He didn't have the ability to come to Jesus himself, so his friends carried him on a mat. Sometimes we don't feel able to come to Jesus, but it is at times like these we can ask our friends to carry us in prayer.

The command Jesus makes in Mark 16 specifically mentions the laying on of hands. When Jesus healed the sick He would sometimes place His hand close to the physical affliction. He touched the skin of lepers, and both the mouth and ears of a deaf, mute man.[260] When the woman who suffered bleeding for twelve years came to Jesus, she touched Him, and as she did, Jesus felt healing power leave Him.[261] Touch can create an empathetic connection but it is also the pattern in the Bible to pray for healing.

---

259. See Luke 5:18.
260. See Matthew 8:2–3; Mark 7:32–37.
261. See Mark 5:30.

238 *I'm Sick, Now What?*

Sometimes when I pray for people's healing, I can feel power travelling through my hands to the place where they need healing. Oftentimes people will report that the area gets hot, and as I pray I can feel this heat increase. Jesus commands us to lay hands on the sick for a reason. (On a practical note, if you are seeking healing for an area that is painful to touch or for an area that would inappropriate to lay hands on directly, it can be best to place your own hands the area and ask those praying to lay hands on top of yours.)

As well as laying hands on the sick, Jesus' followers also had the practice of anointing the sick with oil in order to heal them.[262] Throughout the Bible, oil is used symbolically to represent the presence of the Holy Spirit. Kings,[263] prophets,[264] and priests[265] were anointed with oil to symbolize the Holy Spirit coming upon them. Jesus fulfilled all these offices and was aptly named Messiah, or "the anointed one." To be a Christian is to be a "little" anointed one.

When people pray for your healing by anointing you with oil, it can be a powerful way to symbolize God's presence coming on you. It doesn't matter what oil is used, or how much, as the gesture is symbolic of what is happening in the spiritual realm. For the sake of the sick person, please don't use the method Smith Wigglesworth employed when he started out praying for the sick:

> I had concealed a small bottle in my hip pocket that would hold about half a pint of oil…I pulled the cork out of the bottle, and went over to the dying woman who was laid out on the bed. I was a novice at this time and did not know any better, so I poured all the contents of that bottle of oil over Mrs. Clark's body in the name of Jesus![266]

---

262. See Mark 6:13.
263. See 1 Samuel 9:16; 1 Kings 1:34; and 2 Kings 9:3.
264. See 1 Kings 19:16.
265. Exodus 29:7; Luke 4:18; and Acts 10:38.
266. Quoted in "The Beginnings of His Ministry," SmithWigglesworth.com, http://www.smithwigglesworth.com/life/healing.htm (accessed 29 May 2015).

PRAYER BY CHURCH LEADERS

As well as being prayed for by those close to us, it is also advisable to ask our church leaders to pray. At the end of James' letter, he writes:

> *Is anyone among you sick? Let him call for the elders of the church, and let them pray over him, anointing him with oil in the name of the Lord. And the prayer of faith will save the one who is sick, and the Lord will raise him up.*   (James 5:14–15)

The assumption in this is that you are part of a good, well-functioning church. If you are not currently, maybe one of things God wants to do during your illness is bring you into a healthy spiritual community. I meet a lot of people who have been hurt by people in the church or church leaders, and are no longer part of a congregation, but that is not how it was meant to be. A situation of sickness or pain can motivate you to search out good church leaders who will be helpful to you.

Christianity is not like Buddhism, where you can set up a place of worship at home and worship alone. In the New Testament, believers were always described as being saved and added to a local community. When Paul went around the Mediterranean basin evangelizing, he always gathered new converts into spiritual families.

If you are not part of a church, you not only miss out on regularly connecting with people who in biblical wisdom and pastoral skill could pray into your situation, you also miss out on the chance to be amongst the gathered people of God. There is something quite amazing about God's people gathering together. When all of us who are temples of God gather and worship, we create a larger temple. When this happens, and there is an atmosphere of faith, it often seems easier to hear words of knowledge.[267]

---

267. See 1 Corinthians 12:8, which was written in the context of a gathered church community.

What I love about words of knowledge is that, if they are genuine, they inform a person that God knows his or her situation, and they create a sense of expectation that God has highlighted this for a reason. From experience, if God releases a word of knowledge about particular condition in a particular person, it is usually because He wants to bring about healing. Personally, I find it easier to pray for people who have responded to a word of knowledge, because faith has already risen in the person and myself. But if you are not part of a church, you may miss out on this precious gift.

While I was writing chapter 9 on the importance of faith, I was asked to speak at a student church meeting held on my local university campus. I initially turned down the offer, but I felt God say that I should accept. I spoke on the topic of the chapter, faith, and then gave out a number of words of knowledge that people responded to. A particularly memorable one was for a guy who had a longstanding sporting injury in his right knee. He came to the front in response to the word, and as I commanded the pain to go and the knee to be healed, he instantly felt a change. I got him to bend the knee and then hop on his right leg, and he realized he had been completely healed. For five years he had had reduced function in his knee and now it was fully restored! This may not have happened had he not been part of a church that was open to words of knowledge and praying for healing.

I think there is one caution to be had with James' command. The New Testament is clear that God was not creating only church leaders to be a new priesthood—rather, all of us are to be priests.[268] With this in mind, it would not be wise to call up your church leaders to anoint you with oil as soon as you feel the sniffles of a winter cold. Rather, as a priest yourself, it is important that you try steps one and two before step three.

---

268. See 1 Peter 2:5, 9.

PRAYER BY PEOPLE WITH THE GIFT OF HEALING

A fourth group of people to approach for prayer are people with the gift of healing. Like any of the spiritual gifts mentioned in the New Testament,[269] the gift of healing is given by God to benefit those in the church and assist the church in its mission to reach those who don't yet know Jesus.

I received the gift of healing after I had just qualified as a medical doctor, while attending a church conference. I was sitting in a seminar listening to a topic unrelated to healing. At the end of the teaching, the leader transitioned the seminar into a time of ministry and somebody brought a word of knowledge that God wanted to give the gift of healing to a medical doctor. It seemed I was the only medical doctor in the seminar, and so I went forward for prayer. As I was prayed for, I remember noticing that my hands had an odd sensation come over them. They started to get heavier, and I felt a tingling sensation over my palms. It was as though there was a substance resting on my palms that was not visible. After I was prayed for, I found somebody who was sick. I laid hands on her, and her affliction went away as I prayed. I was elated, but I wasn't really sure what to do next. For some reason I didn't pray for sick people for a while. I would occasionally be in a church meeting when my hands would feel the same way as they did before but then the sensation would go away again and I hadn't, at that point, realized what that signified.

I have since discovered that this is a sign that God wants to use me to heal people. Not everyone with the gift of healing gets a sensation like this. Some people with far more experience than I in praying for the sick receive no sensations. The only way to really know if people have the gift of healing is if they see more people healed than those around them when they pray for healing.

---

269. See 1 Corinthians 12; 14; Romans 12; and 1 Peter 4:10–11.

When people are specifically gifted, they often operate in that gift easily and joyfully. For instance, the gift of administration is one of the spiritual gifts mentioned in the Bible, and you can know the people who have this gift because they can almost effortlessly convert disorder to order, and enjoy doing so. These are often the people who run events or organize conferences. What may look tiring or draining to other people is actually energizing to them, because they are operating in one of their gifts.

Unfortunately, the supernatural gifts often entail such popularity, that a gifted Christian may get caught up in this attention and may misuse or abuse their gift, rather than using it sacrificially. John Wimber, the founder of the Vineyard group of churches, saw many genuine and verifiable healings and had this caution:

> I also visited several healing meetings...and became angry with what appeared to be the manipulation of people for the material gains of the faith healer...dressing like sideshow barkers. Pushing people over and calling it the power of God. And money—they were always asking for more, leading people to believe that if they gave they would be healed.[270]

John Wimber's solution to this abuse of the gift of healing was simple:

> I have made it a matter of policy never to accept gifts for healing. Greed and materialism are perhaps the most common cause of the undoing of many men and women with a healing ministry...When I pray over people for God to release the healing ministry, I always instruct them never to accept money for healing.[271]

---

270. J. Wimber, with K. Springer, *Power Healing* (London: Hodder and Stoughton, 1986), 40.
271. Ibid., 149.

As well as the abuse of the gift of healing, some have even been discovered masquerading as having the gift. I say this all not to cheapen the reputation of the gift of healing, but rather as a caution for Christians to be careful whom we trust when we are in the vulnerable state of being sick. While the gift of healing is a genuine gift that Jesus has given to the church, sadly we need to follow Jesus' instruction to be *"wise as serpents and innocent as doves"* (Matthew 10:16) when assessing people who claim to have this gift. Wise, in being able to identify people who are misusing or only pretending to have a gift of healing, and innocent, by having nothing to do with them. Anybody who gives you the impression that by giving money, your healing will be ensured can quickly be dismissed. The Bible does not link the working of miracles with monetary reward, and, instead, gives examples of people turning down offers to do so.[272]

WHAT SHOULD YOU EXPECT FROM PRAYER?

When you receive prayer for healing a number of things could happen. God may reveal a block to yourself or one of the people praying. There might be someone who God wants you to forgive or He may reveal that your view of Him is unhelpful. Hopefully section two of this book has given you some tools to deal with any blocks that come up. However, you can always ask the Holy Spirit what to do to remove the block. One thing you must not do is ignore it. From experience I know that if God reveals something, He is unlikely to proceed with healing until it is dealt with.

God may also reveal His plan to you. When I was praying for a friend of mine who had been diagnosed with cancer, I felt God tell me He was going to heal him through conventional medicine and that it would take six months. This turned out to be the case, and the knowledge of how it would work out was extremely helpful

272. See 2 Kings 5:16; Daniel 5:17; and Acts 8:20.

to me because I was confident that God had spoken, and it meant I could stop praying for supernatural healing.

God may give wisdom for the next step. God might reveal someone you ought to go to or meet with. It is important to follow through with this, as often God gives us only the first step; once we have completed that, He gives us the next step.

God may start a supernatural healing process. I say "process" because not all healing happens instantly, Instantaneous healing is miraculous, but God also works through healing that happens more slowly—over days, weeks, or months. If this is happening, usually you will be aware that something is happening in your body. There is often warmth or heat in the area you are praying for, and those praying may feel power flowing through their hands. If this happens, I find it is helpful to ask God how long to keep praying for. When I pray for people I will often pause and see if anything has changed. If things are happening quite quickly, I aim to keep praying until all the symptoms leave, but I will stop praying when I sense God saying "stop," even if some symptoms remain.

Nothing may seem to happen. Don't be dismayed by this. This may occur because the people praying are not used to listening to God, or there might be a block between yourself and God that nobody has picked up, or it might simply be part of the spiritual battle. Keep seeking God. (The next chapter addresses what to do if you have been seeking God for years or even decades, seemingly without any change.)

AFTER THE PRAYERS

The important thing is to be honest about whether anything has changed. People who come to pray want to know if something has happened, and it is important to be truthful. It is unhelpful to declare "in faith" that you are healed when you are not. I don't find this practice in Scripture, and it comes across as false rather than truthful. I prayed for someone who had come from a church culture where it was standard to declare healing after having been prayed for. After the prayer, he declared he was healed and got up to leave. I interrupted him and asked him to test whether he had been healed. In complete surprise he realized he had in fact been healed, there and then, to much joy.

If people have prayed with you, ensure that you thank them for their efforts. If nothing has seemed to happen, it can be difficult for the person praying as well as for the one receiving prayer (particularly if they haven't had much experience in praying for sick people). Even if you are feeling down, try and muster up the courage to thank those who gave up time to pray for you. If you have received a partial healing, I think it is definitely worth praying again. Jesus laid hands on a blind man, and after prayer the blind man initially saw people moving like trees. Jesus prayed again and the healing was completed.[273] If nothing has appeared to happen, it is worth asking God if this something you need to persist in. As we saw earlier, Abraham received a son by miraculous birth twenty-five years after he was first promised an heir (more about this in the next chapter!).

If healing seems to have occurred, the first thing to do is test it. If possible, try and do what you couldn't do before. A full healing will lead to pain disappearing and full movement (if the sickness involved a joint). If this has happened, it is important to get the healing verified by a healthcare professional. This is important for a number of reasons. First, if you have truly been healed, a healthcare professional will be able to confirm it. Jesus sent people to the priests (the Jewish doctors of their day) to have healings confirmed.[274] Second, it is important that you see a healthcare professional to oversee any medications you may need to wean off. Some medications are dangerous to stop taking all at once, and so even if you have been healed, it is important that reductions of doses are

273. See Mark 8:22–25.
274. See Luke 17:14.

monitored by an expert. Third, this is a great chance to testify to the healthcare profession that God really heals today, and these healings are medically verifiable. You can use your healing as a chance to talk about the goodness of God in your life.

WHAT IF SYMPTOMS RETURN?

This may seem a strange concept, but it does happen. I prayed for one person who had pain in both knees. When I prayed, I could feel God's healing power on my hands, and the person reported that the pain was instantly leaving. However, that night the person awakened with agonizing pain in both knees again. He rebuked the pain, and it went away and has remained away to this day. What I think happens in these scenarios is that the enemy tries to trick the person into believing that healing has not really happened, and evil tries to recreate the original symptoms. If there has been genuine healing, though, the counterfeit symptoms will be exposed and go away.

What also can happen is that somebody can get healed in the moment, but if the underlying conditions that opened the person up to sickness in the first place aren't dealt with, then the same disease can return. Let me give you a natural example. Imagine somebody with coronary heart disease has had a stent placed in their coronary arteries to keep the arterial hole open and blood flowing through it. If the person doesn't deal with the stress that led to the artery getting blocked in the first place, then it is likely the artery will get blocked again, even with a stent. A similar thing can happen with a spiritual healing; if the underlying condition isn't dealt with, the same problem can reoccur. Review chapters 5 to 8 if you feel symptoms may be returning.

Another way of viewing this is through the lens of faith. A person may have accessed the corporate faith in a meeting to receive healing but didn't have the required individual faith needed to retain the healing. For instance, the first few times that I operated in the gift of prophecy all happened within the context of a corporate atmosphere of faith, but in time I learned to hear God for people outside of these occasions.

If symptoms do return, I suggest that you rebuke the symptoms (out loud) in Jesus' name. If the symptoms still remain, then ask God to reveal if there is an underlying condition that is opening you up to sickness, and then be obedient to what He says to resolve it. If God has initiated a healing, I always take it as a sign that God wants to bring about a full healing. God is our Father, and He doesn't do things to trick us or lead us on. If He starts something, you can ask Him to finish it. If you are under the care of a healthcare professional, I would also advise you to get reassessed if your symptoms return.

Praying for healing, or being prayed for to receive healings, is often quite an emotional process, because the outcome often seems so crucial. We need to remember that physical healing is always secondary to spiritual healing, and if we have received spiritual healing, then regardless of what happens physically, we can rest in the knowledge that God has already completed the greatest miracle.

KEY POINTS

1. Even though Jesus has ascended to heaven, He is still able to heal today; our responsibility is to approach Him for this healing through prayer.

2. We can pray to God for healing by ourselves, with other Christians whom we love and respect, with church leaders, and even from people whom we discern have the gift of healing.

3. Physical healing is not guaranteed on earth, but—if we have received spiritual healing—it is guaranteed in eternity.

CHAPTER 12:

WINNING THE LAST BATTLE

"For richer, for poorer, in sickness and in health"
—*Medieval wedding vows*
Sarum (Salisbury) Diocese, England

Chris had just been ordained as an unsalaried pastor/elder at his local church. He had been married to Jo for seventeen years and had three children, ages eleven, nine, and six. He had been extremely successful in business, and a number of years previously, he had become a Christian. His desire was to have two more children, and one day start a church from scratch.

Suddenly his life took a different direction. Exactly one week after his ordination, Jo developed an unrelenting headache that was so bad, she was admitted to the hospital. The situation became so severe that her doctors induced her medically into a controlled coma, only bringing her out of it two days later. Strangely, the doctors couldn't find the cause of her headaches, and she was in and out of hospital for the next nine months.

After a while she developed a loss of balance, which resulted in difficulty walking. Then she lost coordination in her hands, and then her eyesight deteriorated. All the while her specialists still couldn't find a cause for her symptoms. She eventually lost the ability to speak, became bedridden, and was fed via tube. Finally, she lost her hearing.

Chris went on a forty-day liquid-only fast to plead for his wife's life. People in the church were praying, the pastors/elders laid hands on her and prayed for her, and people with internationally recognized gifts of healing arrived and prayed also. Chris put his business on hold to focus on his wife.

One day, while in his car leaving the hospital, he cried out, "God, what's going on? My wife is lame and blind! Why don't you do something?" To Chris's surprise God answered him, impressing these words in his mind: "I too have a bride who is lame and blind. I will restore your bride. Will you help restore Mine?"

Something changed in Chris in that moment. No longer did God seem distant or unfeeling. Chris now knew that God understood. But God's comment that He would restore His bride left him confused. Did that mean God was going to heal Jo?

Sometime later God said to Chris, "Will you still serve Me if Jo dies?" Chris spent the whole day wrestling with the question. Finally, Chris replied to God that he would but explained that he wouldn't be very happy doing so.

While Jo was in and out of hospital, Chris and his family had many well-intentioned people declare it was God's will that Jo was to be healed. They came up with different things that Chris and the family needed to do, but still Jo deteriorated. Chris felt as though his lack of faith was the reason Jo wasn't getting better.

Not long after, Jo was confirmed to have Creutzfeldt-Jakob Disease (CJD), the human form of BSE (Bovine Spongiform Encephalopathy, or more commonly known as Mad Cow Disease). CJD is incurable, and so, after deteriorating for a further two months, a total of nine months after her initial headache, Jo passed away. All the people who had confidently declared she would be healed were now not so vocal. Chris leaned on the support of a few close friends. At her death God said to Chris, "I have now restored your bride." Chris believed He was referring to Jo being present with Jesus and fully healed.

Two years later, Chris married his current wife, Rachel. On their wedding day, God spoke again to Chris and said, "See, I have again restored your bride. Will you restore Mine?"

A year later Chris and Rachel planted a church in one of the big cities in South Africa. Shortly after starting the church, Rachel gave birth to their first daughter, and eighteen months later, she gave birth to their second. As Chris looked back on events, out of the pain of losing Jo he realized that God had restored him, too. God had even fulfilled his desire to have five children and plant a church.

If you, like Chris, have prayed for healing, for yourself or a loved one, but find there are no signs of improvement, or that the situation even appears to be deteriorating, what should you do next?

PERSEVERE IN SEEKING GOD FOR HEALING

First, if you have prayed for supernatural healing, it is worth noting that results do not always happen instantaneously. Aimee Semple McPherson was a prominent healing evangelist in the 1920s and some follow-up was done with the people who attended her healing services:

> Later in 1921, investigating McPherson's healing services, a survey was sent out by First Baptist Church Pastor William Keeney Towner in San Jose, California, to thirty-three hundred people. Twenty-five hundred persons responded. 6 percent indicated they were immediately and completely healed while 85 percent indicated

252 *I'm Sick, Now What?*

they were partially healed and continued to improve ever since. Fewer than 0.5 percent did not feel they were at least spiritually uplifted and had their faith strengthened.[275]

We can see from this survey that those who reported supernatural healing were fourteen times more likely to experience healing gradually than instantaneously.

Even though much attention is given to instantaneous healing, gradual healing shouldn't be looked down upon. I have heard of longstanding conditions resolving slowly after persistent, daily or weekly prayer, from a person's family, their caregivers, or a regular visiting church leader.

Second, persistence in prayer is important. Jesus teaches us this with two parables: the one about the widow and the judge and the one about a man who wakes his neighbor to ask for bread.[276] In both parables the petitioners don't get their answer straight away, but through persistence they are eventually responded to. In telling these parables Jesus is not comparing God to the unjust judge or the neighbor who isn't that keen to get out of bed. Rather, it's a how-much-more illustration; if even an unbelieving judge or neighbor responds, how much more will God, who loves and cares for His children? Jesus says, *"Will not God give justice to his elect, who cry to him day and night? Will he delay long over them? I tell you, he will give justice to them speedily"* (Luke 18:7–8). Jesus taught these parables to encourage us in persistence. God is keen to answer us, but our job is to persist.

The prophet Daniel found this out when he fasted twenty-one days to hear an answer to a question he had. His answer came very dramatically in the form of an angelic visitation, but the angel told him that his words had been heard the first day he prayed, three weeks earlier. It was only because of a spiritual battle that the answer was delayed.[277] Like Daniel, we don't know what is

---

275. M. A. Sutton, *Aimee Semple McPherson and the Resurrection of Christian America* (Cambridge: Harvard University Press, 2007), 19–20.
276. See Luke 11:5–8; 18:2–8.
277. See Daniel 10.

happening in the spiritual realm when we pray, but we need to remember that God hears our prayers, and until we get an answer, we should persist.

For some people reading this, you may say that you would happily wait three weeks for an answer, but instead it has been years or decades, and you are still waiting. Well, you are in good company. For example, David was only a young boy when the prophet Samuel declared that he would be Israel's next king, but he had to wait until he was thirty years old for this to happen.[278] Similarly, there was a time span of twenty-five years between God promising Abraham he would become a nation, and God opening up Sarah's womb to bear Isaac.[279] Of the heroes of the faith outlined in Hebrews chapter 11, we are told that many of them *"died in faith, not having received the things promised, but having seen them and greeted them from afar"* (Hebrews 11:13).

Like those in Hebrews 11, some of us may receive the healing we request on earth while others of us will only receive our healing on the other side of death. However, whether the people in Hebrews 11 saw what they were promised in their lifetime or not, all of them were commended for their persistence in faith. Dr. Sam Storms, a pastor and former professor of theology, gives this advice:

> We may never know why a person isn't healed. What, then, ought to be our response? In the first place, don't stop praying! Some people find this difficult to swallow… If…you are able to discern, through some prophetic disclosure or other legitimate biblical means, that it is not God's will now or ever to heal you, you may cease asking Him to do so. Otherwise, short of death itself, you must persevere in prayer.[280]

---

278. See 1 Samuel 5:4; 16:1–13.
279. See Genesis 12:1–4; 21:1–6.
280. Sam Storms, "Why God Doesn't Always Heal," Sam Storms: Enjoying God, July 30, 2008, http://www.samstorms.com/all-articles/post/why-god-doesnt-always-heal--2-cor--12:8-10- (accessed 29 May 29, 2015).

Perseverance in prayer is quite normal. Smith Wigglesworth explains it this way: "Everybody has to have testings. If you believe in divine healing you will surely be tested on the faith line. God cannot bring anyone into blessing and into full co-operation with Him except through testings and trials."[281]

PERSEVERE IN SEEKING HOLISTIC HEALING

Third, we must ensure we are seeking God for holistic healing. While we may or may not receive physical healing for our condition, we must remember that is not the only healing open to us. Matt Chandler, whose story we read in chapter 10, said this:

> I am an excellent studier and researcher, and before all this began, I would say a decent man of prayer; but I learned after they told me I only had two to three years left that I knew much more about God than I actually knew Him. The bulk of my sanctification through this ordeal has been the birth of a deep desire for intimacy with our great God and King.[282]

Sickness often brings to the surface things buried deep within us that may not have come to our attention had we remained well. God cares deeply about these things and wants us to be healed of anything that holds us back from connecting with Him, and flourishing in life. During his battle with cancer, John Wimber, founder of the Vineyard churches with an extensive healing ministry, spoke candidly about struggling with depression at the same time.

---

281. Quoted in "The Beginnings of His Ministry," SmithWigglesworth.com, http://www.smithwigglesworth.com/life/healing.htm (accessed 29 May 2015).
282. Matt Chandler, "Don't Waste Your Cancer: Interview with Matt Chandler," *Tabletalk*, July 1, 2011, http://www.ligonier.org/learn/articles/dont-waste-your-cancer-interview-matt-chandler/ (accessed 29 May 2015).

Depression in those who are sick long-term, or in those who have been diagnosed with severely disabling conditions, is very common, but God wants to meet us in our depression and be a support to us. The Psalms are a good source of help to us in this area. If you are feeling depressed it may be helpful to follow some of the psalmists and use their template to speak out your feelings to God. God is able and willing to engage with us if we bring our thoughts and feelings to Him.

As Chris discovered, whatever our emotional state, if we cry out to God, He will answer us. When Elijah was burned out and depressed to the point of requesting death, when he called out, God engaged with him. As well as providing for his physical needs, God corrected some wrong thoughts Elijah had, encouraged him with a newer perspective, gave him a new commission, and provided him with a successor to carry on his current role.[283] Once Elijah engaged with God, God carried out a very holistic healing.

If God were to answer you in the way He answered Elijah, what would you want Him to do for you? What would holistic healing look like for you?

When I was working as a hospital doctor, for a short time I carried around a small book of World War I poems. As a person who had grown up in a time of relative peace, I was horrified to discover what those particular soldiers went through. During the First World War the media was very different to what it is today; back home, the public was buoyed by descriptions of the valor and the glory of war. But the death of nineteen thousand Allied soldiers on the first day of the Battle of the Somme told a different story. Nineteenth-century war tactics met twentieth-century weaponry; as they were ordered to climb out of their trenches and charge toward the enemy, the soldiers were mowed down by machine guns. If they were not killed during these suicide missions, they were deafened by unceasing shellfire or poisoned by nerve toxins.

---

283. See 1 Kings 19:1–18.

Many soldiers were shot by their own side for attempting to flee the battle scene. Back home, survivors were greeted as heroes, but rather than celebrating their return, many were suffering from post-traumatic stress, feeling like victims of torture. Surrounded by people who couldn't even begin to imagine what they had gone through, some of the artistically gifted among them turned to poetry to communicate the horrors that they had experienced.

One of my professors was quite surprised when he saw me reading the poems, wondering why, in a profession that saw much death, I would want to read about more of it in my free time. I don't think I made the connection at the time, but looking back I think it gave me a window into what some of my patients were experiencing. My patients, like soldiers, were in the thick of a battle. Relatives and friends would do their best to sympathize, but only somebody who was also caught up in the battle, or somebody who had come through the other side, would ever be able to truly empathize and understand what they were feeling. As a doctor I was even further from understanding this than my patients' friends and relatives, but the war poems gave me the beginnings of an insight, and the ability to form a small connection.

Connections during times of suffering are crucial. Romans chapter 8 tells us that God wants to, and is able to, connect with us at our deepest level. It reveals God as Someone who prays on our behalf, even expressing the groans we feel deep in our spirit. In the times in our lives when words have failed us, when we have long since found any way of expressing our torment, Paul's letter to the Roman church tells us there is One who knows and who understands.

God is not distant. Jesus knows the agony of crying out in pain and anguish while heaven remains silent. He knows the injustice of reaping what others have sown, and what it feels like to have His closest friends abandon Him at His time of need. If you have had these experiences during your sickness be assured that there is One who can truly empathize and relate. There is One who has been in the battle and come through the other side.

On the cross Jesus cried out: *"My God, my God, why have you forsaken me?"* (Mark 15:34). In doing so He was teaching us to pursue God during our pain, even when heaven seems silent. The huge difference, though, is that while the Father didn't answer Jesus, He now will answer us. The separation that Jesus experienced was because of the sin we committed. Through the cross, Jesus took on our alienation from God and gave us His perfect connection. Jesus was forsaken, so that we didn't have to be. Once we place our trust in Him, Jesus then ensures that there is nothing that can separate us from God's love.[284]

So, as you persist, know that you have access to a God who will help you. When you can no longer groan, know that you have a God who will groan on your behalf. Know that you have a God who is not distant and remote but a God who can relate to what you have been through. A God that stood His ground and came through the other side.

WHAT SHOULD WE DO IF WE ARE FACING DEATH?

Unless Jesus returns in our lifetime, even if we are healed, all of us will face death at some point, and it is important that we prepare for this—not just legally, by preparing a will, etc., but also spiritually.

While doing my pre-med degree I worked as nursing assistant at my local hospital so that I could become familiar with the world I was about to enter. It was far from glamorous; my job mostly consisted of giving out meals and assisting patients to bathe and wash, but I learned a lot. On one occasion, when I was looking after a man who was quite sick, the patient cried out loudly that he was dying while still in sin. Because he was in a bay with three other patients, I drew the curtain round his bed and spoke to him about his distress. I discovered he was Roman Catholic, and he

284. See Romans 8:35.

was requesting a priest come to him so that he could take his confession and, according to his belief, die with his sins absolved.

Whether he had taken a sudden turn for the worse that had taken him off guard or whether he had longstanding sins that he had kept secret, I do not know, but what was certain is that he didn't feel spiritually prepared for death.

It doesn't have to be this way for us. Whether death is imminent or not expected for decades, we can all be in a place where we are spiritually prepared for death. To be best prepared I believe we need peace in three sets of relationships.

The first relationship is between God and us. My Catholic patient didn't feel at peace with God, and this was deeply troubling and disturbing as death approached him. The first level of peace between God and us is plain from Scripture. We need to know that God has forgiven our sins and that we have been adopted as His child. As a pastor, this is one of the most important things that I probe for when caring for people spiritually. To do so I tend to ask one of two questions: Is Jesus in charge of your life? Or, if you were to die today, would you be with Jesus? The first question is quite helpful because the Bible tells us that it is impossible to call Jesus Lord (Master) except by the Holy Spirit.[285] I take the second question on the basis that Jesus could promise to the thief next to Him on the cross that they would be together after His death.[286]

When I was at university, I went to a Christian festival that included going into the city of Manchester, UK, and engaging with people about their views on faith. One person I met was a Buddhist priest who was also out on the street engaging with people, but promoting Buddhism.

It turned out to be a very interesting conversation because he told me how much he admired Jesus as a powerful god. As he waxed lyrical about Jesus, a thought came to my mind, wondering

---

285. See 1 Corinthians 12:3.
286. See Luke 23:43.

if he actually knew Jesus. I had heard of Jesus appearing to many Muslims in dreams and connecting with them, and I thought maybe Jesus had reached out to Buddhists as well. So, I said to him "You say that Jesus is very powerful, so is He your Boss or Lord?" There was a palpable change in the atmosphere and he took a step back and said, "Oh, no. He is not *my* god." He went on to say that because the Holy Spirit had blocked Paul from going to Asia, he believed that the Buddha was the god for Asians and Jesus had been given a different region.[287] I didn't pay too much attention to his argument because I was so struck by how clear things were in the spiritual realm. It doesn't matter how much somebody may admire Jesus or say He is great—in the spiritual realm, either Jesus is Lord of somebody's life or He isn't.

If you honestly can't say that Jesus is your Lord or you are not sure if you would be with Him were you to die now, then it is of great importance that you act on that realization. Jesus' offer of life eternal is real and true, but it costs the right to be in charge of our life here and now. If we want to be rescued by Jesus from the negative consequences of His coming judgment, we have to repent of our sin, give up control of our life and then allow Him to be in charge. I asked Jesus to take charge of my life when I was very young—I had seen enough of God in my parents that I just seemed to know that giving Him charge would be a better option than trying to find my own way through life. It was only later as I regularly took charge back from Him that I realized how rebellious I was and how in need of rescuing I was. And that realization has only gotten deeper the older I get, but I can now answer those two questions with great authority: yes, Jesus is in charge of my life, and yes, when I die I will be with Him. If you can't say those two things, is there anything stopping you from saying sorry for missing God's mark and asking Jesus to be in charge of your life, right now?

---

287. See Acts 16:6. What the priest failed to understand is that three chapters later, we are told *"all the residents of Asia heard the word of the Lord"* (Acts 19:10).

Why not use this prayer as a template: *Jesus, I am sorry that I have lived in rebellion to Your ways. I have acted selfishly, placing my needs above You and others. Please forgive me specifically for* _____. *I now ask You to be in charge of my life and that You teach me how to live for You and Your kingdom. Amen.*

Accepting Jesus as Lord and Savior is the essential first step for us to have peace between God and us; however, like any other relationship, we still need to deal with issues that may arise along the way. That is why I wrote section two of this book, to assist people in deepening their connection with God. If we would like to be spiritually prepared for death, then it would make sense that we deal with any relational blocks between God and us.

Flowing from being at peace with God should come a desire to be at peace with others, as well. It is also necessary to restore these relationships before death as much as you are able to. Palliative care physician Ira Byock wrote a book called *The Four Things That Matter Most.* He writes about what dying patients say is important to say to loved ones before it's too late. The four phrases are: (1) please forgive me; (2) I forgive you; (3) thank you; and (4) I love you.[288]

Many people put off trying to restore relationships, telling themselves they will do it one day, but for many that day never comes, and they find themselves approaching death without a further opportunity.

Have a look at that list and ask yourself: (1) who do I need to ask forgiveness from? (2) who do I need to speak to and say that I forgive them? (3) who do I need to thank, whom I haven't expressed thanks to? and (4) who needs to hear me say that I love them?

Don't wait until it is too late. Can I suggest that you act on your realizations and start making a plan to carry out each of your answers? You will derive great benefit from doing so, and you might be surprised by how people react.

---

288. Ira Byock, *The Four Things That Matter Most* (New York: Free Press/Simon & Schuster, 2004).

Finally, as well as making peace between ourselves and God, and making peace between ourselves and those around us, a third set of relationships we can assist in bringing peace to is between God and those who don't know Him.

In his book *Crafted Prayer*, Graham Cooke recounts when his dying friend George asked him if God had told Graham whether he was going to be healed or not.[289] Graham, put on the spot as George's loved ones surrounding his bedside looked up at Graham and waited for an answer, responded by telling him what he felt God had said, simply saying: "Have a great death." The atmosphere in the room chilled while George processed these words, but after a moment he declared to Graham, "Grae, I'm going to have the greatest death you have ever seen." Subsequently George wrote down the names of twenty-four people he knew who weren't believers and invited them all to visit him. As George told them about Jesus' offer of reconciliation, twenty-three of them became Christians. As he died, the twenty-fourth, seeing the peaceful smile on George's face, knelt down on the floor and accepted Jesus as his Savior and Lord.

George may not have received healing on earth, but ultimately it didn't matter because he already had the most important healing. Happily, he used his death to ensure others experienced the same. Is there anything stopping you from being like George, in life and death?

REST IN THE KNOWLEDGE THAT SPIRITUAL HEALING IS GUARANTEED

The cross shows us that we are called to persist, but Jesus' cry, "*It is finished*" (John 19:30), shows us we are also called to rest; to rest in the knowledge that Jesus has done it all. Seen in the light of an eternity of healing, even if sickness takes our earthly bodies, we

289. Graham Cooke, *Crafted Prayer* (Grand Rapids, MI: Chosen Books/Baker Publishing, 2004), 47.

can rest in the knowledge that this time of sickness will only represent an infinitesimally small fraction of our future experience of complete health. In the infinitely greater scheme of God's promise of eternal health, our sickness affects us for just a moment. We can rest now in the guarantee of a new body that will never experience sickness or decay.[290]

The apostle Paul knew this well. With a back scarred from one hundred and ninety-five lashes, with a body that had been bludgeoned by gangs armed with clubs and pummeled with heavy rocks, with a memory that had experienced three shipwrecks and near-drownings, and with an eyesight that seemed to be failing, he was still able to say: *"We are hard pressed on every side, but not crushed; perplexed, but not in despair; persecuted, but not abandoned; struck down, but not destroyed"* (2 Corinthians 4:8–9 NIV).

After originally persecuting the church, Paul was transformed into someone who was persecuted himself, voluntarily suffering so that others could become disciples of Jesus. During his mission to reach out to those who didn't know Jesus, he was regularly hungry and thirsty and suffered exposure from the cold. He was the victim of robbers and wild animals and yet despite this he was able to respond: *"We are…not crushed…not in despair…not abandoned…not destroyed."* While chained and incarcerated for Christ, he sang of God's goodness.[291] It is not surprising that he could say to the Philippian church that he had discovered the secret of contentment in whatever circumstance he found himself in.[292]

Is this possible, for all of us? That even when our body is failing, we can access the deep peace and contentment that Paul experienced? Paul told the Corinthian church, *"Though our outer self is wasting away, our inner self is being renewed day by day"* (2 Corinthians 4:16). John Wimber experienced this wasting away in the midst of spiritual success. Thousands were healed through

---

290. See 1 Corinthians 15:42–44.
291. See Acts 16:25.
292. See Philippians 4:11.

his ministry and yet, at age sixty-three, his outer body gave way to cancer. John G. Lake taught thousands to access God's supernatural healing, but at the age of sixty-five he suffered a stroke and his body passed on. Smith Wigglesworth saw huge numbers of incredible miracles, but he looked on while his wife and son died long before him, and while he could pray for others to be healed, his own daughter remained deaf her whole life.

Paul carries on: *"For this light momentary affliction is preparing for us an eternal weight of glory beyond all comparison, as we look not to the things that are seen but to the things that are unseen"* (2 Corinthians 4:17). The joy described by Paul doesn't come to us through looking at what is happening in the earthly realm. The more real our understanding of heaven and eternity are, the less dominant the things of this world are to us.

All around us there is a lust for health at all costs. If this world was all there is, then you and I should join them, giving everything we have to maintain our health and happiness—but it isn't! There is a realm beyond this world.

Brother Yun, a Chinese house church leader, is an eminent example of living beyond this world. His story is told in the book *The Heavenly Man*.[293] Yun became a Christian at age sixteen and was first imprisoned at age seventeen in a freezing cold prison cell. During his arrests and imprisonments he was repeatedly beaten (sometimes with electric batons) and tortured. His crime: he was preaching the gospel. During his final imprisonment the prison guards broke both his legs. Why did Brother Yun endanger his life and endure such terror? The only credible answer is that he had a hope greater than any pain in this world—that he had an eternal perspective.

King Nebuchadnezzar must have thought that Daniel's three friends were similarly brash and foolhardy when they accepted

---

293. See Brother Yun with P. Hattaway, *The Heavenly Man: The Remarkable True Story of Chinese Christian Brother Yun* (Grand Rapids, MI: Kregel, 2002).

death by incineration rather than bow down to his statue.[294] But they didn't see it as risky. King Nebuchadnezzar was asking them to swap obedience to an eternal heavenly master for obedience to a temporary earthly master; to swap the affections of a God who would love and care for them forever for the disregard of a ruthless dictator who cared nothing for them. But to everyone else not in the know, it must have sounded strange when they said, "*Our God whom we serve is able to deliver us…But if not, be it known to you, O King, that we will not serve your gods or worship the golden image that you have set up*" (Daniel 3:17–18). In Babylon, gods were worshipped for what they could do for you in this life, but Shadrach's, Meshach's and Abednego's God gave provision not just for this life, but also the next.

As you look to the certainty of your future healing and the joy of knowing God now, friends may scorn or look bemused at your faith in a God that may not have seemed to have done a great deal for you, but they don't know what we know—that our healing is guaranteed. Truly we can say to them, "Our God is able to heal us…But if not, we will continue to worship Him."

In 1940, Germany was on the ascendancy in the Second World War and had pushed back the Allied forces from Belgium, through France, right to the French coastline. The British Prime Minister Winston Churchill called it a "colossal military disaster."[295] Facing either the annihilation or the capture of the three hundred and fifty thousand troops, one British officer sent a telegram back to London declaring the army's intent. The telegram had just three words: "But if not." In an age of biblical literacy, the meaning was instantly recognizable. The army's determination and defiance in the midst of such dire circumstance accessed the compassion of a nation, and, even, it seems, the heart of God.

---

294. See Daniel 3:1–18.
295. Winston Churchill, "Wars are not won by evacuations," 4 June 1940, House of Commons. Cited in Winston S. Churchill, *Never Give In! The Best of Winston Churchill's Speeches* (New York: Hyperion, 2003).

Still to this day, historians discuss why Adolf Hitler hesitated and ordered the Nazi army to not deliver the killer blow. His hesitation gave enough precious time for the Allied troops to gather at the nearest port, Dunkirk. Back in the UK, a national day of prayer was held, followed by hundreds of British civilian shopkeepers, fishermen, and owners of pleasure boats piling into their little crafts and travelling through the night with the British Navy as it crossed the English Channel. While the majority of the soldiers were able to board the Navy ships at the port, many others were ferried by the civilian boatmen who risked their own lives to do so. Because of this combined military and civilian effort, over a period of nine days 338,226 soldiers were miraculously brought back safely to Britain. Many historians mark it as one of the key turning points of the war.

The greatest words of faith we may ever declare might be, "But if not." If we utter them in our most desperate situation they will act as a rousing declaration that all of heaven cannot help but applaud. Are you willing to persist in seeking God to the point of "But if not"? To the point of staring complete loss in the face and going on to say, "My God is able to heal me…But if not, I will still worship him"?

If you are, then, by God's grace, you can confidently say, "*For I am sure that neither death nor life, nor angels nor rulers, nor things present nor things to come, nor powers, nor height nor depth, nor anything else in all creation, will be able to separate [me] from the love of God in Christ Jesus our Lord.*"[296]

KEY POINTS

1. If you have prayed for supernatural healing, remember that results do not always happen instantaneously and it is important to persist in prayer.

---

296. Romans 8:38–39.

2. Even if we are healed, all of us will die eventually. We can prepare spiritually for death by seeking peace between God and us, between others and us, and between God and others.

3. Even if sickness takes our earthly bodies, God can grant us eternal healing; and from the perspective of eternity, our experience of sickness will only be a tiny fraction of our total existence.

APPENDIX:

PRESENCE OF THE GIFT OF HEALING IN OPERATION IN EVERY CENTURY OF THE CHURCH

There is extensive proof of God's miraculous healing in every century of the church since Christ's death and resurrection. Below is a sampling of Christians' accounts of miraculous healing experiences.

FIRST CENTURY

The New Testament writings name specifically Peter, John, Paul, Barnabas, and Ananias, all following Jesus' example and healing the sick. The gospels tell of the twelve and the seventy-two seeing healings occur when they went out on missions, and in James' letter, believers are encouraged to pray for the sick who are in the church.

SECOND CENTURY

JUSTIN MARTYR (A.D. 100–165)

Justin was a prominent apologist for the Christian faith, arguing for the Roman Emperor Antonius to bring a halt to the persecution of Christians. He founded his own philosophical school to promote Christianity in Rome, but fell into a dispute with another philosopher and was beheaded by the Roman authorities. Subsequently, the concept of martyrdom was named after him. In *Second Apology* (A.D. 153), Justin Martyr wrote about the continuation of the gift of healing:

> For numberless demoniacs throughout the whole world, and in your city, many of our Christian men exorcising them in the name of Jesus Christ, who was crucified under Pontius Pilate, have healed and do heal, rendering helpless and driving the possessing devils out of the men, though they could not be cured by all the other exorcists, and those who used incantations and drugs.[297]

IRENAEUS (A.D. 130–202)

Irenaeus was bishop of Lyons in Gaul (modern-day France) and was also a powerful apologist, fighting particularly against the heresy of Gnosticism. He believed in the continuation of supernatural healing and in his *Against Heresies* (A.D. 185) he details many instances of supernatural healings, and even a number of people being raised from the dead.[298]

---

297. Justin Martyr, *The Second Apology of Justin*, vol. 1 of *Ante-Nicene Fathers* (Peabody, MA: Hendrickson, 1999), Chapter VI.
298. Irenaeus, *Against Heresies*, vol. 1 of *Ante-Nicene Fathers* (Peabody, MA: Hendrickson, 1999).

THIRD CENTURY

ORIGEN (A.D. 184–253)

Origen was a prominent theologian from Alexandria, Egypt. His father was martyred during an outbreak of persecution but his mother protected him from the same fate. In his book *Against Celsus* (A.D. 250), Origen wrote about the gifts of the Spirit being in operation in the church, and said that those with healing gifts were producing "many cures."[299]

NOVATIAN (A.D. 200–258)

Novatian was famous for separating from the Church of Rome and forming his own church, over the issue of readmitting people who had denied their faith during persecution. Other than this difference, his church had the same theology and practice as the Roman church and continued into the seventh century. In chapter 29 of his *Treatise of Novatian Concerning the Trinity* (A.D. 270), Novatian wrote of healings and wonderful works being done in the Lord's church everywhere:

> This is He who places prophets in the Church, instructs teachers, directs tongues, gives powers and healings, does wonderful works, offers discrimination of spirits, affords powers of government, suggests counsels, and orders and arranges whatever other gifts there are of charismata; and thus make the Lord's Church everywhere, and in all, perfected and completed.[300]

---

299. Origen, *Against Celsus*, vol. 4 of *Anti-Nicene Fathers*, trans. Frederick Crombie (Peabody, MA: Hendrickson Publishers, 1999).

300. Novatian, *Treatise of Novatian Concerning the Trinity*, vol. 5 of *Ante-Nicene Fathers*, trans. Robert Ernest Wallis (Peabody, MA: Hendrickson, 1999), 29.

FOURTH CENTURY

AUGUSTINE (A.D. 354–430)

Augustine was bishop of Hippo (modern day Algeria, Africa) but is famous for his theological works, *Confessions and City of God*, which are still widely read today. He is often called the "Father of Western Christianity." Although originally not a believer in the continuation of the supernatural gifts, Augustine was compelled by the genuine healings he saw around him, and in the last section of The City of God he wrote about the miraculous healings that he had witnessed personally, including a blind man receiving sight.[301]

HILARION (A.D. 291–371)

Hilarion was born in Gaza (modern day Palestine). When he was fifteen his parents died, and he gave away his inheritance to his family to the poor and lived an ascetic life in the desert. After twenty-two years of this hermitic lifestyle, he became famous and was sought out for wisdom and prayer. Jerome, in his *Life of Saint Hilarion* (A.D. 390), recounts a number of healings that occurred during Hilarion's ministry, including successfully praying for a barren woman to have a son and a woman blind of ten years receiving instantaneous sight.[302]

---

301. Augustine, *The City of God*, vol. 2 of *Nicene and Post-Nicene Fathers, First Series*; trans. Marcus Dods (Peabody, MA: Hendrickson,, 1999), 8.
302. Jerome, *The Life of Saint Hilarion*, vol. 6 of *Nicene and Post-Nicene Fathers, Second Series*; trans. W. H. Fremantle (Peabody, MA: Hendrickson, 1999), 305–306.

FIFTH CENTURY

PATRICK OF IRELAND (A.D. 387–461)

Patrick was a Scottish missionary to Ireland who saw many of its warring tribesmen become Christians. In *The Life and Acts of Saint Patrick*, a biography written by Jocelin, a twelfth-century Scottish monk, it reads:

Under this most sanctified rule of life did he shine in so many and so great miracles that he appeared second to no other saint. For the blind and the lame, the deaf and the dumb, the palsied, the lunatic, the leprous, the epileptic, all who labored under any disease, did he in the name of the Holy Trinity restore unto the power of their limbs and unto entire health; and in these good deeds was he daily practised. Thirty and three dead men, some of whom had many years been buried, did this great reviver raise from the dead, as above we have more fully recorded. And of all those things which so wondrously he did in the world, sixty and six books are said to have been written, whereof the greater part perished by fire in the reigns of Gurmundus and of Turgesius. But four books of his virtues and his miracles yet remain, written partly in the Hibernian, partly in the Latin language; and which at different times four of his disciples composed.[303]

---

303. Jocelin, *The Life and Acts of St Patrick*, trans. James O'Leary (New York: P. J. Kenedy, 2006 [1880]), 186.

SIXTH CENTURY

COLUMBA (A.D. 521–597)

Columba was an Irish missionary to Scotland. He founded a number of abbeys, including an abbey on the Isle of Iona, which was the dominant Christian center in Scotland for centuries. Adomnán, a relative and also a monk, wrote the account of Columba's life in *Vita Columbae* ("Life of Columba," written as three books). In book two, Adomnán describes many healing miracles occurring through Columba, even people who had died being brought back to life.[304]

AUGUSTINE OF CANTERBURY (D. A.D. 604)

Augustine was an Italian missionary who was sent to England to evangelize the then-pagan nation. At that time England was made up of a number of kingdoms and Augustine went first to King Aethelberht, who had recently married the Christian daughter of a French king. King Aethelberht, and many others, became Christians and this led to the founding of the English church, with Augustine as its first archbishop (of Canterbury). Robin Mackintosh, in his book on Augustine, states there was a "notable ministry of healing and miracles that took place through Augustine and his monks, and that these wonders, healing in diseased and broken bodies as well as souls, were an authentic witness to the gospel for their time."[305]

---

304. Adomnán, *Life of Columba* ed. and trans. A.O. Anderson and M. O. Anderson (Oxford: Oxford University Press, 1991, 2nd ed.).
305. R. Mackintosh, *Augustine of Canterbury: Leadership, Spirituality and Mission* (London: Canterbury Press, 2013), 149.

SEVENTH CENTURY

CUTHBERT (A.D. 634–687)

Cuthbert lived in Northern England but was of Celtic origin. He was the bishop of Lindisfarne, in the kingdom of Northumbria (modern day Northern England). In book four of his biography, *Vita Sancti Cuthberti* ("Life of St. Cuthbert"), a number of healings are recorded, including healing an infant from the plague and a boy from paralysis.[306]

EIGHTH CENTURY

BEDE (A.D. 673–735)

Bede was an English monk, author and scholar, based in Northern England. He translated many Latin and Greek early church writings, enabling his fellow Anglo-Saxons to have access to them. In his *Ecclesiastical History of England*, Bede writes of healings frequently, including healing somebody of blindness and raising an earl's (English lord) servant back to life. [307]

NINTH CENTURY

ANSGAR (A.D. 801–865)

Ansgar was archbishop of Hamburg-Bremen, in Germany, and missionary to Sweden and Denmark, where he founded many churches and monasteries. This led to him to being known as the "Apostle of the North." Adam of Bremen, in his *Deeds of the Archbishops of Hamburg-Bremen*, states that at one time Ansgar

---

306. Bertram Colgrave, ed. and trans., *Vita Sancti Cuthberti* (Cambridge: Cambridge University Press, 1940).
307. Bede, *A History of the English Church and People*, vol. 6, trans. Leo Sherley-Price (Harmondsworth, UK: Penguin, 1955).

visited a hospital in Bremen daily, and "healed very many by his speech and by his touch."[308]

TENTH CENTURY

LUKE OF HELLAS (D. A.D. 946)

Luke lived an ascetic life out of devotion to God. He founded a monastery and church in Steiri, in mainland Greece, which remains to this day. In *The Life and Miracles of St. Luke of Steiris*[309] Luke is reported to have performed many miracles, including healing sicknesses.

ELEVENTH CENTURY

ANSELM OF CANTERBURY (1033–1109)

Anselm, originally from Arles (modern-day France), was a philosopher and, as Archbishop of Canterbury, head of the English church. He was famous for being the originator of the ontological argument for God, but Eadmer, in his biography of Anselm, tells us he was also famed as a worker of wonders. For instance, at times he miraculously produced food for his companions, and he once instantly healed a boy with a pain in his groin.[310]

TWELFTH CENTURY

BERNARD OF CLAIRVAUX (1090–1153)

---

308. Adam of Bremen, *History of the Archbishops of Hamburg-Bremen*, ed. and trans. Francis J. Tschan (New York: Columbia University Press, 1959).

309. C. L. & W. R. Connor, trans., *The Life and Miracles of St. Luke of Steiris* (Brookline, MA: Hellenic College Press, 1994).

310. Eadmer, *Life of St Anselm*, ed. and trans. R.W. Southern, (Oxford: Oxford University Press, 1972).

Bernard was the abbot of Clairvaux Abbey, France, and a gifted leader, rapidly expanding the Cistercian Monastic Order into many countries. His monasteries emphasized the reading and reflection of Scripture, empowered by the Holy Spirit. Bernard was also known for moving in the gifts of the Spirit. Watkin Wynn Williams, in his biography of Bernard, tells of a time when Bernard laid hands on a boy who was lame and saw him healed instantly.[311]

THIRTEENTH CENTURY

DOMINIC OF OSMA (1170–1221)

Dominic was a Spanish monk and founder of the Dominican Order, a movement of travelling preachers. He was well-educated but when a famine hit Spain, he sold his furniture, manuscripts, and clothes to raise money to feed the poor. Reverend Alban Butler in his book *The Lives of the Saints* recounted that Dominic performed a "great number of miracles," including three accounts of people being brought back to life after they had died. [312]

FRANCIS OF ASSISI (1181–1226)

Francis grew up in a wealthy family in Assisi, Italy. After conversion, he renounced his wealth and lived among the poor. He wore only a rough garment tied by a rope, and travelled barefoot to preach the gospel. As others joined him, he founded the Franciscan Order, which grew rapidly. Many miracles were linked to Francis, including the healing of physical and mental illnesses. In chapter 25 of his book *The Little Flowers of St. Francis*, Ugolino Brunforte

---

311. Watkin Wynn Williams, *St. Bernard of Clairvaux* (Manchester: Manchester University Press), 274.
312. Alban Butler, Rev., *The Lives of the Fathers, Martyrs, and Other Principal Saints* (Dublin: James Duffy, 1866; Bartleby.com, 2010, accessed 10 June 2015).

reports that Francis came across a leper who was bitter toward God. Francis washed the skin of the leper and it was miraculously healed, and the leper then repented of all his bitterness.[313]

FOURTEENTH CENTURY

SERGIUS OF RADONEZH (1314–1392)

Sergius was a Russian monk who founded Holy Trinity Monastery, north of Moscow. He and his followers went on to found around forty monasteries, based on a principle of simplicity and manual labor. Sergius was associated with the miraculous, and his followers reported a time when he prayed for a boy who died of sickness, and the boy came back to life.[314]

FIFTEENTH CENTURY

MARTIN LUTHER (1483–1546)

Martin was born in Saxony (modern-day Germany), and was famous for initiating the Protestant Reformation, and founding the Lutheran churches. Initially he was an Augustinian friar, then ordained as a Catholic priest, followed by becoming a professor of theology. On becoming disillusioned with the difference in practice of the Catholic Church from what he saw in the Bible, he posted ninety-five objections on a church door, which eventually led to his excommunication.

In response to a letter asking for instruction in dealing with severe depression Martin Luther wrote:

---

313. Ugolino Brunforte, *The Little Flowers of St. Francis*, ed. and trans. W. Heywood (New York: Vintage Spiritual Classics, 1998).
314. Serge Zenkovsky, *Medieval Russian's Epics, Chronicles, and Tales* (New York: E. P. Dutton, 1974).

If the physicians are at a loss to find a remedy, you may be sure that it is not a case of ordinary melancholy. It must, rather, be an affliction that comes from the devil, and this must be counteracted by the power of Christ with the prayer of faith. This is what we do and what we have been accustomed to do, for a cabinet maker here was similarly afflicted with madness and we cured him by prayer in Christ's name...when you depart, lay your hands upon the man again and say, "These signs shall follow them that believe; they shall lay hands on the sick, and they shall recover." Do this three times, once on each of three successive days. Meanwhile let prayers be said from the chancel of the church, publicly, until God hears them....Other counsel than this I do not have.[315]

COLETTE OF CORBI (1381–1447)

Corlette was born in Picady, France. She was a member of the Poor Clares, an order founded by Francis of Assisi. She went on to found eighteen convents that focused on a life of austerity and regular fasting. Sabine Baring-Gould, in his book *The Lives of the Saints*, wrote this:

> "I am dying of curiosity to see this wonderful Colette, who resuscitates the dead," wrote the Duchess of Bourbon, about this time. For the fame of the miracles and labours of the carpenter's daughter was in every mouth...After having spent two years at Vevey, Colette went to Nozeroy, to the princess of Orange, and remained with her till 1430. Philip the Good, Duke of Burgundy, recalled Colette to Flanders, where she founded several houses, and glorified God by many miracles.[316]

---

315. Martin Luther, *Luther: Letters of Spiritual Counsel*, ed. and trans. by Theodore G. Tappert (Vancouver, BC: Regent College Publishing, 2003), 52.
316. Sabine Baring-Gould, *The Lives of the Saints*, vol. 3 of 16 (The Project Gutenberg, March 1, 2015).

SIXTEENTH CENTURY

GERASIMOS OF KEFALONIA (1506-1579)

Gerasimos was born in to a wealthy family in Greece and was ordained as monk at Mount Athos. After spending twelve years in Jerusalem, he returned to Greece and founded a monastery on the island of Kefalonia, which became a center of charity and a place of care for the poor. In a history of his life, recorded by the Orthodox Church in America, we are told he was "granted a miraculous gift: the ability to heal the sick and cast out unclean spirits."[317]

SEVENTEENTH CENTURY

GEORGE FOX (1624-1691)

George Fox was the founder of the Religious Society of Friends (Quakers). George saw many people healed in response to his prayers. John Banks (1638–1710) testified to George's healing gift in his journal:

> About this time [1677], a pain struck into my shoulder, which gradually fell down into my arm and hand, so that the use thereof I was wholly deprived of; and not only so, but the pain greatly increased both day and night and for three months I could neither put my clothes on or off myself, and my arm and hand began to wither, so that I did seek to some physicians for cure, but no cure could I get by any of them; until at last as I was asleep upon my bed in the night time, I saw in a vision I was with dear George Fox; and I thought I said unto him, "George, my faith is such, that if thou seest it thy way to lay thy hand upon my

---

317. "Venerable Gerasimus the New Ascetic of Cephalonia," Orthodox Church in America, http://oca.org/saints/lives/2014/10/20/103007-venerable-gerasimus-the-new-ascetic-of-cephalonia (accessed 10 June 2015).

shoulder, my arm and hand shall be whole throughout."...
in Lancashire, where there was a meeting of Friends...
some time after the meeting, I called [George] aside into
the hall, and gave him a relation of my concern...he turned
about and looked upon me, lifting up his hand, and laid
it upon my shoulder, and said, "The Lord strengthen
thee both within and without." And so we parted, and
I went to Thomas Lower's of Marsh Grange that night;
and when I was sat down to supper in his house, immediately, before I was aware, my hand was lifted up to do its
office, which it could not for so long as aforesaid; which
struck me into great admiration, and my heart was broke
into true tenderness before the Lord, and the next day I
went home, with my hand and arm restored to former use
and strength, without any pain. And the next time that
George Fox and I met he readily said, "John, thou mended,
thou mended;" I answered, "Yes, very well in a little time."
"Well," said he, "give God the glory."[318]

In 1672, while visiting in the Carolinas, George Fox wrote this
account in his journal:

And many people of the world did receive us gladly and
they came to us at one Nathaniel Batts, formerly governor of Roanoke, who goeth by the name of Captain Batts;
who hath been a rude desperate man. He came to us and
said that a captain told him that in Cumberland, George
Fox bid one of his friends to go to a woman that had been
sick a long time, and all the physicians had left her, and
could not heal her. And George Fox bid his friend to lay
his hands upon her and pray for her, and that George Fox's
friend did go to the woman, and did as he bade him, and
the woman was healed at that time. And thus Captain

318. Quoted in Edmund Goerke, *The Gift of Healing in the Life of George Fox*,
http://www.quakerinfo.com/healing1.shtml (accessed 10 June 2015).

Batts told me, and spread it up and down the country among the people. And he asked of it, and I said many things had been done by the power of Christ.[319]

EIGHTEENTH CENTURY

JONATHAN EDWARDS (1703–1758)

Jonathan Edwards was an American Puritan pastor, philosopher, and theologian during the Great Awakening. He had a keen mind, graduating from Yale as valedictorian, and is regarded as one of America's greatest intellectuals. He wrote,

> In the former part of this great work of God amongst us, till it got to His height, we seemed to be wonderfully smiled upon and blessed in all respects. It was the most remarkable time of health that ever I knew since I have been in the town….We ordinarily have several bills put up, every Sabbath, for sick persons; but now we had not so much as one for many Sabbaths together.[320]

JOHN WESLEY (1703–1791)

John Wesley graduated with a theology degree from Oxford University, and brought about a spiritual renewal while working as a pastor in the Church of England. He went on to cofound with his brother the Methodist Church, which has grown to eighty million adherents today. In 1741, he wrote in his journal:

> Friday 8th May, I found myself much out of order. However, I made shift to preach in the evening: but on Saturday my bodily strength quite failed, so that for

---

319. George Fox, *The Journal of George Fox*, vol. 2 (Cambridge: Cambridge University Press, 1911), 234.
320. Jonathan Edwards, "A Narrative of Surprising Conversions" in *On Revival* (Carlisle, PA: Banner of Truth, 1999), 69.

several hours I could scarce lift my head. Sunday 10th. I was obliged to lie down most part of the day, being easy only in that posture. Yet in the evening my weakness was suspended while I was calling sinners to repentance. But at our love-feast which followed, beside the pain in my back and head, and the fever which still continued upon me, just as I began to pray, I was seized with such a cough that I could hardly speak. At the same time came strongly into my mind, "These signs shall follow them that believe." I called on Jesus aloud, to "increase my faith" and to "confirm the word of his grace." "While I was speaking, my pain vanished away; the fever left me; my bodily strength returned; and for many weeks I felt neither weakness nor pain. Unto thee, O Lord, do I give thanks." [321]

NINETEENTH CENTURY

THE SALVATION ARMY (1865–PRESENT)

William and Catherine Booth founded the Salvation Army in London, and it quickly expanded to Austria, Ireland, and the United States. Today, it has one and a half million adherents and operates in 126 countries. In the 1880s, the Salvation Army held healing campaigns in Canada, and Captain Payne, in Stratford, Canada, reported that "the deaf hear, the lame walk and the leprous sinners are cleansed."[322] In 1886, the Salvation Army magazine *The War Cry* (New Zealand) reported a testimony of Wilhelmina Ross, who had been paralyzed for sixteen years, and who had been supernaturally healed.[323] In 1902, General Booth

321. John Wesley, *Journal of John Wesley* (Christian Classics Ethereal Library: http://www.ccel.org/ccel/wesley/journal.vi.iv.v.html, accessed 10 June 2015).
322. James William Opp, *The Lord for the Body*, (Montreal, QC: McGill Queen's University Press, 2005), 84.
323. C. A. Fulton, "Letter to the Editor: Divine Healing," *The War Cry* (New Zealand), July 3, 1886.

wrote a memorandum, clarifying the church's position on healing: "God does, when He sees that He can thus glorify Himself and benefit men, go out of His ordinary course in healing the sick in answer to the prayer of faith."[324]

TWENTIETH AND TWENTY-FIRST CENTURY

THE PENTECOSTAL MOVEMENT (1906–PRESENT)

Most people place the birth of the Pentecostal Movement in Los Angeles in 1906, with the Azusa Street Revival. William J. Seymour led worship meetings that consisted of very diverse congregants, from the extremes of rich and poor and a mixture of races (which was very counter-cultural for the time period). Seymour taught on the baptism of the Spirit as a separate event to conversion with the accompaniment of spiritual gifts, particularly the gift of tongues. Thousands came to take part in the meeting and many missionaries were sent out from there. For instance, in the first two years the movement had spread to an astonishing fifty nations, and the resultant Pentecostal Movement now numbers 279 million adherents.[325] Belief in the continuation of the gift of healing is one of the movement's key doctrines, and Pentecostals report regular physical healings. The 1950s led to the popularity of healing evangelists, who preached in large tent meetings, teaching and demonstrating physical healing.

THE CHARISMATIC MOVEMENT (1960–PRESENT)

As the Pentecostal Movement affected those in traditional denominations, a second movement arose, called the Charismatic

---

324. General William Booth, *Faith Healing: A Memorandum* (London: International Headquarters of The Salvation Army, 1902), 9.
325. Pew Forum on Religion and Public Life, "Global Christianity," December 19, 2011, "Global Christianity: A Report on the Size and Distribution of the World's Christian Population," 67.

Movement. This was characterized by the operation in the more miraculous spiritual gifts, including the gift of healing, but with less of an emphasis on speaking in tongues, than in Pentecostalism. Because the movement arose within the traditional churches, the theology and culture of charismatics tended to be quite different from Pentecostals. As time went on, many charismatics left the traditional churches they were part of and established "newer" churches. Over five hundred million people are associated with either a newer charismatic church or Pentecostal church, making the combined Pentecostal/Charismatic Movement the fastest growing church movement in the world today.[326]

---

326. Ibid.

ABOUT THE AUTHOR

Dr. Andrew Butterworth is a pastor at Junction Church, Johannesburg, South Africa. Trained as a doctor at the University of St. Andrews and then the University of Manchester, with an additional degree in public health, Dr. Butterworth worked in various hospitals around the United Kingdom's Greater Manchester area before transitioning to public health and church ministry in South Africa, where he now lives with his wife, Michelle.